# The Silver Drawing Test
## *and* Draw a Story

MW00354735

# The Silver Drawing Test *and* Draw a Story

Assessing Depression, Aggression, and Cognitive Skills

## RAWLEY SILVER, EdD, ATR-BC, HLM

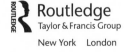

Routledge
Taylor & Francis Group

New York   London

Routledge
Taylor & Francis Group
270 Madison Avenue
New York, NY 10016

Routledge
Taylor & Francis Group
2 Park Square
Milton Park, Abingdon
Oxon OX14 4RN

© 2007 by Rawley Silver
Routledge is an imprint of Taylor & Francis Group, an Informa business

Printed in the United States of America on acid-free paper
10 9 8 7 6 5 4 3 2 1

International Standard Book Number-10: 0-415-95534-3 (Softcover)
International Standard Book Number-13: 978-0-415-95534-8 (Softcover)

No part of this book may be reprinted, reproduced, transmitted, or utilized in any form by any electronic, mechanical, or other means, now known or hereafter invented, including photocopying, microfilming, and recording, or in any information storage or retrieval system, without written permission from the publishers.

**Trademark Notice:** Product or corporate names may be trademarks or registered trademarks, and are used only for identification and explanation without intent to infringe.

**Library of Congress Cataloging-in-Publication Data**

Silver, Rawley A.
    The Silver drawing test and draw a story : assessing depression, aggression, and cognitive skills / Rawley Silver.
        p. cm.
    Includes bibliographical references and index.
    ISBN 0-415-95534-3 (pb)
    1. Psychological tests for children. 2. Draw-A-Story. 3. Depression in children--Diagnosis. 4. Aggressiveness in children--Diagnosis. 5. Cognition--Testing.    I. Title.
        [DNLM: 1. Psychological Tests. 2. Depressive Disorder--diagnosis. 3. Aggression. 4. Cognition. 5. Risk Assessment. 6. Child. WS 105.5.E8 S587s 2007]

RJ503.7.P76S55 2007
618.92'891653--dc22                                                                                  2006028342

**Visit the Taylor & Francis Web site at**
**http://www.taylorandfrancis.com**

**and the Routledge Web site at**
**http://www.routledgementalhealth.com**

For Ed, with love


The words or the language, as they are written or spoken, do not seem
to play any role in my mechanism of thought. The psychical entities
which seem to serve as elements in thought are . . . in my case, the
visual and some of the muscular type. Conventional words or other
signs have to be sought for laboriously only in the second stage.

—Albert Einstein


The scientific search for truth and the human search
for understanding belong together.

—Jacob Bronowski

# Contents

◇　◇　◇

## SECTION I  DRAW A STORY: SCREENING FOR DEPRESSION AND AGGRESSION

# Contents

## SECTION II THE SILVER DRAWING TEST: DRAWING WHAT YOU PREDICT, WHAT YOU SEE, AND WHAT YOU IMAGINE

# Contents

## SECTION V   APPENDICES

# Contents

# List of Figures

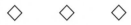

# List of Figures

# List of Figures

# Foreword

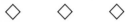

It is a privilege to introduce the reader to this book by one of the most respected authors in the art therapy profession. Dr. Rawley Silver's career has been a long and distinguished one. Her published writing spans four decades and her contributions to the body of research in the field have been recognized and appreciated. She has been the recipient of the Research Award of the American Art Therapy Association four times. The scope and depth of Dr. Silver's research are impressive. She enlists the cooperation of therapists worldwide, skillfully incorporates their findings, and constantly updates her work. Her creative and scientific approach to research has helped build credibility for the relatively young profession of art therapy.

To fully understand and appreciate Dr. Silver's work, one must consider the context in which it was developed, as well as the person who created it. Dr. Silver participated in the formation of the art therapy profession, presenting her work at the earliest conferences. In 1962 when she was working with deaf and hearing impaired children in New York City her first article on the benefits of art making for deaf children appeared in a professional journal. Her contributions extended beyond direct services, research and writing. During those early years she organized two traveling exhibitions of the art of deaf children that were circulated by the Smithsonian Institution. Illustrated catalogs for both shows were created. Her dedication and energetic efforts helped expand community awareness of the creativity and intelligence of these children.

# Foreword

In 1978 her first book was published. *Developing Cognitive and Creative Skills through Art* contains some of the foundations for her later work. The book is replete with examples of children's art that demonstrate Dr. Silver's ability to inspire her young clients' trust and artistic creativity. Theory is presented clearly and her contentions are unfailingly supported with data.

Stemming primarily from her work with the deaf, Dr. Silver went on to create the tests that comprise this book. As the reader will see, today they are used with many different client populations. Therapists who are new to these tests may be pleasantly surprised by how receptive clients are when offered this testing material. Simple, unthreatening and stimulating to the imagination, the tests are usually well received even by highly resistant individuals. The stimulus drawings inspire metaphorical art that is rich in content and the accompanying stories yield a wealth of material to explore with clients. Many interesting examples of drawings and stories are included in this book.

Rawley Silver, in her life and work, provides us with an example of the artist/scientist practitioner. In the tradition of other art therapy pioneers, such as Margaret Naumburg, Edith Kramer, and Janie Rhyne, she believes that art is at the heart of the professional practice of art therapy. Her work attests to the fact that one does not have to sacrifice the "art part" of the practice of art therapy in order to take a scientific approach. The integration is as much a part of who she is as of what she writes. An accomplished artist herself, Rawley Silver continues to paint, draw and exhibit her work. Her confidence in the future of the profession is summarized in these remarks from the 1998 film *Rawley Silver: Art Therapist and Artist*:

> Art therapists bring something no other group can and that is the perception, sensitivity, and empathy that comes with understanding drawings. Art therapy has a future and a valuable contribution to make. I'd like to see it continue to draw on both the scientific community and the art community as only art therapy can. That's the way I hope it will go.

With the publication of this book, Dr. Silver has once again contributed to the likelihood of just that. Readers seeking a balanced perspective that integrates creativity and research can feel confident that Rawley Silver speaks with great integrity and with authority derived from many years of experience. I expect that this book will be welcomed and appreciated by the art therapy community as well as by experienced practitioners in other human services fields. It will join Dr. Silver's other books as an enduring classic in the art therapy literature.

**Christine Turner, ATR-BC, LPC, NCC**
*Chairperson, Department of Graduate Studies in Art Therapy Counseling*
*Marylhurst University, Marylhurst, Oregon*

# Acknowledgments

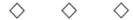

The studies reviewed in this book could not have been carried out without the help of many. Their assistance is gratefully acknowledged. They include art therapists who served as judges in the studies of scorer reliability and art therapists and teachers who volunteered to administer the drawing tasks and/or score responses.

In addition to the art therapists and others whose studies are discussed in this book, I wish to thank Georgette d'Amelio, MS; Victoria Anderson-Schwacher, MA; Doris Arrington, MA, ATR-BC; Janice Bell, MA; Nancy Benson, Allison Berman, MA, ATR; Andrea Bianco-Riete, MA, ATR-BC; Jennifer Blackmore, MA, ATR-BC, MS; Eldora Boeve, MA; Sherry Carrigan, MA, ATR-BC; Felix Carrion, MA, ATR; Hope Larris Carroll, MA, ATR; Lin Carte, MA, ATR-BC; Fran Chapman, MA; Linda Chilton, MA, ATR; Bette Conley, MA, ATR; Sylvia Corwin, MA; Peggy Dunn-Snow, PhD, ATR-BC; Cheryl Earwood, MA, ATR-BC; Joanne Ellison, MA, ATR-BC; Patricia English, MA, ATR; Raquel Farrell-Kirk, MA, ATR-BC; Melinda Fedorko, MA, ATR-BC; Betty Foster, MA; Cyrilla Foster, MA, ATR; Phyllis Frame, MA, ATR; Enid Shayna Garber, MA, ATR-BC; Elizabeth Gayda, MA; Madeline Ginsberg, MA, ATR-BC; Maryanne Hamilton, MA, ATR-BC; Robin Hanes, MA, ATR; Karen Hayes, MA; David Henley, MA, ATR-BC; Eileen McCormick Holzman, MA, ATR-BC; Ellen Horovitz, PhD, ATR-BC;

# Acknowledgments

Patricia Isis, MA, ATR-BC; Judith Itzler, MA, ATR; Lynn Jamison, MA, ATR; Beth Kean, MA; Alexander Kopytin, MD, CMS; Janeen Lewis, MA, ATR; Jared Massanari, PhD; Maggie McCready, MA; Kate McPhillips, MA, OTR; Madeline Masiero, MA, ATR-BC; Eva Mayro, MA, ATR; Carol McCarthy, MA, ATR; Sally McKeever, MA; Sr. Dorothy McLaughlin, MA, ATR-BC; Christine Mercier-Ossorio, MA, ATR; Yetta Miller, MA, ATR; Linda Montanari, MA, ATR, LMFT; Constance Naitove, MA, ATR; Ruth Obernbreit, MA, ATR; JoAnne O'Brien, MA, ATR; Bernice Osborne, MA; Norma Ott, MA; Carol Paiken, MA; Sara Jacobs Perkins, MA; Linda Jo Pfeiffer, PhD, ATR-BC; Marcia Purdy, MA, ATR; Lillian Resnick, MA, ATR-BC; Michelle Rippey, MA, ATR-BC; Kimberly Sue Roberts, MA, ATR; Louise Sandburg, MA, ATR; Sr. Miriam Saumweber, MA, ATR; Patricia Schachner, MA; Andrea Seepo, MA, ATR; Vlada Sventskaya, CPS; Helen Svistovskaya, MD; Joan Swanson, MA; Niru Terner, MA, ATR; Sr. Mary Tousley, MA, ATR; Christine Turner, ATR-BC; Kristen Vilstrup, MA, ATR-BC; Robert Vislosky, PhD, ATR; Mary Waterfield, MA, ATR; Jules C. Weiss, MA, ATR-BC; Phyllis Wohlberg, ATR; and Shelley Zimmerman, ATR-BC.

I would also like to thank the psychologists who provided the statistical analyses. They include Madeline Altabe, PhD; Brooke Butler, PhD; John L. Kleinhans, PhD; Beatrice J. Krauss, PhD; and Claire Lavin, PhD.

Finally, I want to thank the anonymous children, adolescents, and adults who created the drawings and stories reprinted here. I am deeply grateful for their participation.

**Rawley Silver, EdD, ATR-BC, HLM**

# Chapter 1

# Introduction

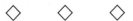

Much has happened since *Three Art Assessments* was published in 2002. New studies have found that the Draw a Story assessment can be used to identify children and adolescents at risk for violent behavior as well as for depression, and two subgroups of aggression have emerged: predatory and reactive. In addition, there have been new studies of the Silver Drawing Test of Cognitive Skills and Emotion by practitioners in Russia, Thailand, and the United States, and scoring guidelines have been made more precise.

To include these new findings, I streamlined the Draw a Story assessment and the Silver Drawing Test but more had to go—condensing the third assessment, Stimulus Drawings and Techniques, into a single chapter of techniques for developing cognitive skills, and moving its stimulus drawings to appendix C.

The original purpose of the Draw a Story (DAS) assessment was to identify children and adolescents with masked depression. Their responses to the drawing task provided access to thoughts and feelings that were inaccessible through words, and recent studies have found that their responses can serve to identify those who may harm others as well as themselves.

The Silver Drawing Test (SDT) evolved from a theory that drawings might be used to bypass the language deficiencies of deaf children, to evidence that responses to its drawing tasks can be used not only to assess cognitive skills that escape detection on language-oriented tests of intelligence and achievement but also provide access to the fantasies of typical children and adolescents. The SDT has been used to assess emotional as well as cognitive strengths and weaknesses, and has been used with adults as well as children and adolescents.

DAS and the SDT use stimulus and response drawings as the primary channel for receiving and expressing ideas. They are based on the premise that drawings can bypass verbal deficiencies and serve as a language parallel to words, that emotions and cognitive skills can be evident in visual as well as verbal conventions, and that even though traditionally identified and assessed through words, they can also be identified and assessed through images.

The stimulus drawings are line drawings of people, animals, places, and things. Some are explicit, while others are ambiguous in order to elicit personal associations with past experiences. The assessments provide different sets of stimulus drawings but present the same Drawing from Imagination task, which asks respondents to choose two stimulus drawings, imagine something happening between the subjects they choose, draw what they imagine, add titles or stories, and—whenever possible—to discuss their responses so that meanings can be clarified.

Respondents tend to perceive the same stimulus drawings differently, and alter them in subtle ways, intentionally and unintentionally. Some choose subjects that represent themselves or others in disguise. Others use drawings to express fear or anger indirectly or fulfill wishes vicariously, using symbols and metaphors.

Both assessments include 5-point rating scales that range from strongly negative to strongly positive in emotional content, self-image, and use of humor. In addition, the SDT provides 5-point scales for assessing cognitive skills, and includes three tasks: Drawing from Imagination, Predictive Drawing, and Drawing from Observation. Each task has been designed to assess one of the three concepts said to be fundamental in mathematics and reading, as discussed in chapter 6.

## Why the Assessments Were Developed and How They Evolved

Initially, the assessments were developed in experimental art classes for children with hearing impairments. My interest in deafness began when I was temporarily deafened myself in midlife. Painting had been my vocation, and, after recovering, I volunteered to provide studio art experiences to deaf students in a school that did not have an art teacher. The children assigned to my class were emotionally disturbed as well as deaf, and since only one could lip-read or speak and I did not know how to sign, we communicated, at first, through pantomime. Then I tried a quick sketch of my family, gesturing an invitation to sketch in reply. A tall girl responded with a sketch of her mother, father, and sister, then added herself isolated by a tree and the smallest in her family. A boy whose father had disappeared drew himself, his siblings, mother, and beside her, a picture on the wall.

Although most of the students loved to draw, a few were reluctant or shy, and I offered them simple line drawings as possible subjects. The sketches they chose most often were offered to others, and eventually became stimulus drawings in the assessments.

The first assessment published was *Stimulus Drawings and Techniques* in 1981, followed by *The Silver Drawing Test* in 1983. Most responses to the Drawing from Imagination task expressed thoughts and feelings, but a few were fantasies about suicide. Subsequent studies found that these responses, scoring 1 point, correlated significantly with responses by children and adolescents who had been hospitalized for clinical depression, and *Draw a Story: Screening for Depression* was published in 1987. The assessments were revised during the 1990s, and in 2002, revised again into a single volume, *Three Art Assessments*.

## Theoretical Background

Neuroscientists, using magnetic resonance imaging scans, have been tracking mirror neurons, a fundamental brain mechanism. The function of mirror neurons may be to detect mental states and empathize with the behaviors of others, enabling one individual to understand the emotions, intentions, and actions of another (Gallese, Keysers, & Rizzolatti, 2004). This mind-reading ability works through feelings, not conceptual reasoning. Our brains have the capacity to link "what *I* do and *I* feel" directly with what someone else does and feels. It responds when we experience emotions or purposeful actions, and when we observe the same emotions or actions in others. The empathy circuits light up and the brain internalizes representations of the external world. These mirror neurons could explain why watching media violence may be harmful, why some people like pornography, and why people respond to music and the visual arts (Blakeslee, 2006).

These findings raise questions that relate to the studies reported here: Do stimulus and response drawings activate mirror neurons? Do stimulus drawings prompt respondents to empathize with the subjects they choose and project emotion into their responses? Do their drawings enable us to sense a respondent's motivation and state of mind?

Other neuroscientists have been examining relationships between the visual brain and the arts. According to Semir Zeki, the preeminent function of the visual brain is to acquire knowledge about the world, and achieves this knowledge by selecting essentials and discarding what is superfluous, whereas artists have the ability to "abstract the essential features of an image and discard redundant information, essentially identical with what the visual areas themselves have evolved to do" (1999, p. 17).

Visual artists have expressed similar ideas. Ching Hao, a painter in tenth-century China, wrote that painters "should disregard the varying minor details, but grasp their essential features," and try "to fathom the significance of things and to grasp reality" (1948, pp. 84, 92). In addition, Hindu artists spoke of capturing and conveying the "*rasa*" or essence, according to Ramachandran and Hirstein (1999).

Even though these neuroscientists cite the observations of Hindu artists, they exclude the experiences of practicing artists from their studies, as Amy Ione (2000) points out, and they also fail to provide empirical evidence.

Like mature artists, unskilled children, adolescents, and adults seem to reveal essences in the subjects they choose and the feelings they express in responding to the drawing task, as well as in their use of humor.

How do our brains process humor? Neuroscientists can make patients cry or smile by stimulating particular regions of the brain, but have difficulty making them laugh, and puns are processed in the left hemisphere, nonverbal jokes in the right. Do mirror neurons enable us to perceive and respond to the various kinds of humor—morbid, disparaging, resilient, playful—expressed through drawings?

Other neuroscientists have been studying the relationships between thoughts and feelings. According to LeDoux (1996), cognition and emotion work together rather than separately, and both involve symbolic representations. Lane and Nadel (2000) note that they are linked inextricably; and Damasio (1994) proposes that human reasoning consists of several brain systems working in concert, that emotions are one of the components, and that, contrary to traditional opinion, emotions are involved in decision making and just as cognitive as other percepts.

Psychologists have used drawings to assess emotions and measure intellectual maturity for more than 50 years. The House, Tree, Person Test (Buck, 1948) and Kinetic Family Drawings (Burns & Kaufman, 1972) assess emotional indicators. The Draw-a-Man Test (Goodenough & Harris, 1963) measures intellectual maturity. The Human Figure Drawing Test (Koppitz, 1968) assesses level of intellectual development as well as emotions. The Torrance Test of Creative Thinking (Torrance, 1984) measures fluency, flexibility, originality, and elaboration.

For more than 40 years, art therapists have demonstrated that drawings can be used to assess and enhance emotional well-being. Some art therapists present unstructured tasks to encourage spontaneity whereas others specify what to draw (Cohen, 1986; Gantt & Tabone, 1998; Kramer, 1971; Lachman-Chapin, 1987; Levick, 1989; Malchiodi, 1997, 1998; Rubin, 1987, 1999; Shoemaker, 1977; Ulman, 1987).

Draw a Story and the Silver Drawing Test are based on the premise that limiting choices can stimulate creativity, and that structuring need not inhibit spontaneity. If we offer choices within boundaries, and encourage respondents to feel free to make final decisions, structured tasks can provide emotional support, particularly when drawing is a novel experience. In addition, the assessments are concerned with content rather than form; with meanings rather than colors, shapes, or other physical attributes; with visual and verbal brain functions; and the mysteries of humor.

## Quantitative and Qualitative Findings

This volume presents its findings in two forms: quantitative and qualitative. The quantitative findings are based on groups large enough for statistical analyses; they include experimental and control groups, rating scales, normative data, and studies of reliability and validity. The qualitative studies are based on subgroups too small for statistical analysis, and on individuals: the behaviors, histories, and response drawings of particular children, adolescents, young adults, and senior adults.

I believe that both forms are essential. Without both, the wealth of information that emerges about individuals and small groups vanishes within groups large enough for statistical analyses. On the other hand, without empirical evidence, findings remain speculations.

Other observers have recognized and defined the value of both forms of knowledge. Jacob Bronowski (1973), a scientist at the Salk Institute, has suggested that the scientific search for truth and the human search for understanding belong together, that science has a way of formalizing its language so that it can be persuasive and constantly checked, whereas art and literature carry many messages, not one, and speak for our most secret thoughts and feelings.

Fluornoy has noted that the scientific intellect analyzes, abstracts, and generalizes, and when it deals with particular objects, dissolves their particularity; but it is just this individuality that is the exclusive interest of art (in Allen, 1967).

Stern (1965) has distinguished between the analytical and the intuitive; the artist's knowledge is intuitive, subjective, and poetic, "an immediate beholding of essences" (p. 42). It can be experienced but not explained, and is contrary to the scientist's knowledge, acquired through objective analysis. Nevertheless, we can study movement both ways, by floating in the stream ourselves or by timing the passage of a stick as it floats past certain points on shore.

## How the Book Is Organized

Section I, "Draw a Story: Screening for Depression and Aggression," consists of four chapters. Chapter 2 includes guidelines for administering and scoring, together with examples of scored responses. Chapter 3 reviews findings of reliability and validity. Chapter 4 reviews new findings about aggression and depression. Chapter 5 concludes this section with ways that various practitioners have used DAS to assess children, adolescents, and adults with and without emotional disturbances, as well as those who experienced abuse, delinquency, brain injuries, or other disorders.

Section II, "The Silver Drawing Test: Drawing What You Predict, What You See, and What You Imagine," presents similar findings about the SDT, along with the addition of a chapter of normative data. It reviews recent and previous findings of studies that used the assessment for access to the cognitive skills, emotions, and attitudes of individuals and groups with hearing impairments, brain injuries, and learning disabilities, as well as children, adolescents, young adults, and senior adults with no known impairments.

Section III, "The Use of Both Assessments by Practitioners in Florida and Abroad," presents updated reports by art therapists who have been using both assessments with students in Florida, as well as reports by practitioners in Australia, Brazil, Russia, and Thailand.

Section IV, "Developmental Techniques and Concluding Observations," includes studio art techniques for developing cognitive skills, and a chapter of discussion and conclusions.

Section V, "Appendices," provides testing materials for the SDT and DAS assessments in appendixes A and B, and the original 50 stimulus drawings in appendix C.

# Section I

# Draw a Story: Screening for Depression and Aggression

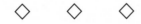

# Chapter 2

# Background

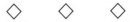

There is an urgent need to identify children and adolescents who may harm others or themselves. Suicide has become a leading cause of death, and antisocial behavior is increasing. The aim of the Draw a Story (DAS) assessment is to identify those at risk. After summarizing its background, this chapter presents guidelines for administering its assessment and scoring responses.

## Why DAS Was Developed and How It Evolved

A few children drew suicidal fantasies when responding to the Drawing from Imagination task of the Silver Drawing Test (see appendix A), raising questions whether drawings could be more revealing than face-to-face interviews, and whether the task might be useful in screening for masked depression. Because certain stimulus drawings seemed to elicit these negative fantasies, I included them in a new set of stimulus drawings, and presented them first to children in elementary schools, and then to adolescents and adults.

As it turned out, our studies found that strongly negative responses to the drawing task, scoring 1 point on the emotional content scale, are associated with clinical depression among children and adolescents. Responses by adults are more guarded and tend to score 3 points (ambivalent, ambiguous, or unemotional). Studies of reliability and validity also were undertaken, and the Draw a Story assessment was published (Silver, 1988a, 1988b). It was revised in 1993, and again in 2002.

Recently, studies of children and adolescents with histories of aggressive behavior found that their responses to the DAS task also have distinctive characteristics that can be quantified: strongly negative fantasies scoring in point on the emotional content scale, combined with strongly positive self-images, scoring 5 points on the self-image scale (Earwood, Fedorko, Holzman, Montanari, & Silver, 2004). The findings suggested that DAS responses could be used to screen for aggression as well as depression, and subsequent studies have expanded these findings (Silver, 2005).

## Aggression

Incidents of aggression occur frequently in schools. Although some schools address them effectively, others are overwhelmed with responsibilities, and potentially violent students may be overlooked. Teachers have reported that bullies victimize only about 15% of their students, but students tend to disagree. MacNeil (2002) cites studies that found 50% of students reported being bullied, and 65% had witnessed bullying. In addition, students in urban, suburban, and rural schools reported similar rates. The number of seriously injured children nearly quadrupled from 1986 to 1993 (Bok, 1998). Other children inflicted a substantial proportion of their injuries, and homicide has become the second leading cause of death for Americans aged 15 to 45. Although preventive programs focus on students with histories of violent behavior, angry but quiet students may be overlooked, as noted in Pfeiffer (2005).

Fischer and Watson (2002) have identified two characteristics that predict the development of physical violence toward others: harsh physical punishment in the family, and inhibited temperament of the child. They distinguish between shyness and inhibited temperament, and suggest two factors that predict aggressiveness in children with inhibited temperaments: fearfulness in general, and low self-esteem.

Connor (2002) defines appropriate aggression as adaptive, its social values changing as societies change, and suggests that there is a continuum from appropriate to inappropriate aggression. He defines inappropriate aggression as maladaptive and dysfunctional, an angry reaction to real or perceived danger that may include depression. Some depressed children, unlike adults, do not appear sad or suppress angry feelings. They tend to misinterpret and overreact, blame others, and expose themselves to danger. Their aggressiveness emerges earlier in life, and may result from abuse, harsh parental discipline, or family instability.

Connor also suggests four subtypes of aggressive behavior: offensive, defensive, relational, and harmful to oneself. Offensive aggression is characterized by unprovoked attacks with intent to benefit the aggressor. It is motivated by reward, such as dominance, territory, food, or the acquisition of objects. It tends to arouse little emotion and is reinforced by success and by social role models. He cites studies that found correlations of aggression with positive expectations and social dominance. Offensive aggressors tend to be callous and unable to empathize; they gang up on victims and use force to have their way. They also tend to hide their aggressiveness and protect themselves from injury.

Defensive aggression, as defined by Connor, is an angry reaction to real or perceived danger, and arises in response to threats or frustration. It produces intense arousal and is hypervigilant and impulsive. Its intent is to harm the source of frustration, to inflict injury or pain rather than benefit the aggressor, and to defend against threat. It may include depression, social withdrawal, anxiety, fear, and/or confrontations with others, such as fighting or defying authority, and is associated with peer rejection and exposure to violence.

Connor defines relational aggression as harming a victim's relations with others, and aggression that is harmful to one's self as suicidal ideation. Relational aggression did not seem to appear in the findings reported here, but suicidal ideation appeared frequently.

## Depression

Studies of major depressive disorders have found that children and adolescents show an increased risk for homicidal as well as suicidal ideation, according to Connor (2002), who also notes that depressed children and adolescents do not suppress their anger—unlike depressed adults, who tend to suppress angry feelings.

A study of 100 suicides by children found that a majority had manifested antisocial behavior (Shaffer & Fisher, 1981). Pfeffer (1986) distinguished suicidal from non-suicidal children by their feelings of hopelessness and the wish to die. Some children mask depression with antisocial behavior, expressing fantasies of violence, explosions, annihilation, and death with bad outcomes for principal subjects (McKnew, Cytryn, & Yahries, 1983). Three major patterns of depression were cited by Beck, Rush, Shaw, and Emory (1979): negative views of self, negative views of the future, and a tendency to interpret one's experiences in a negative way. These patterns have appeared frequently in responses to the Drawing from Imagination task.

## The Use of Humor

Ziv (1984) has proposed that humor serves various functions. Aggressive humor serves to hide aggressive feelings by enabling us to punish others and feel superior in a socially acceptable way. Humor also enables us to defend against fears by laughing at them and providing a sense of mastery. It helps us face reality, relieve tension, avoid depression, and deny dangers by making them appear ridiculous. Self-disparaging humor serves to win sympathy and reduce anxiety.

Vaillard (2002) has emphasized mature forms of humor, noting that they permit us to look directly at what is painful, laugh at our own misery, vent angry feelings, and loose blunt arrows against others. Under stress, however, they may change to less mature defenses, such as passive-aggressive behavior (expressing aggression toward others indirectly) or acting out (directly expressing unconscious wishes or impulses).

## Administering the DAS Assessment and Scoring Responses

The DAS assessment can be presented individually or to groups of examinees. Individual administration is recommended for those who are being examined clinically and for children younger than seven years of age. The age range is from five years to adult. There is no time limit, but the task is usually finished within 10 minutes. Classroom teachers, as well as art therapists, psychologists, and other clinicians, have administered and scored the DAS assessment successfully without special training.

Figure 2.1 presents the DAS Form A set of stimulus drawings, which should be used only for pre- and posttesting. Figure 2.2 presents the second set, Form B, which is provided for any other purpose, such as developing cognitive skills, or obtaining additional responses so that patterns in emotional content, self-image, or the use of humor may emerge. The full test booklet may be found in appendix B, together with other testing materials.

Provide each respondent with a copy of the DAS test booklet. When testing examinees who may have difficulty reading the directions, say,

> I believe you will enjoy this kind of drawing. It doesn't matter whether you can draw well. What matters is expressing your ideas. Here are some drawings of people, animals, places, and things. Choose two picture ideas and imagine a story, something happening between the pictures you choose.
>
> When you are ready, draw a picture of what you imagine. Show what is happening in your drawing. You can make changes and draw other things, too.
>
> When you finish drawing, write a title or story. Tell what is happening and what may happen later on.

If a respondent chooses to draw different subjects or simply copies the stimulus drawings, do not intervene unless you feel the instructions were misunderstood.

After drawing has started, minimize discussions and avoid interruptions, including your own. As respondents finish drawing, ask them to add titles or stories and fill in the blanks on the lines provided. If respondents have difficulty writing, ask if they would rather dictate their stories to you; and if they do, write their exact words on the lines provided.

It is important to be supportive and encouraging. The experience should be pleasurable and an opportunity for quiet reflection. Erasers are provided so that responses can be revised.

Whenever possible, discuss the drawings individually so that meanings can be clarified. It is important to make respondents feel it is safe to express thoughts and feelings. If they use symbols or metaphors, use them too. For example, if the drawing is about a cat and mouse, you might ask, "Can you tell me how the cat (or mouse) feels or what it is thinking? What has happened and what may happen later on?" Be alert for verbal clues, such as personal pronouns or the subjects of sentences. Metaphorical dialogues often provide opportunities to introduce healthier adaptations or alternative solutions.

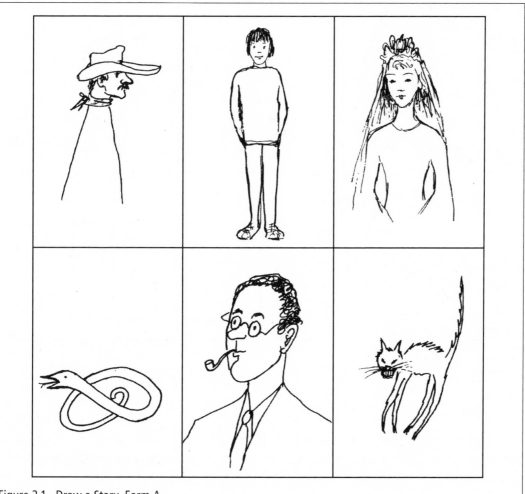

Figure 2.1. Draw a Story, Form A.

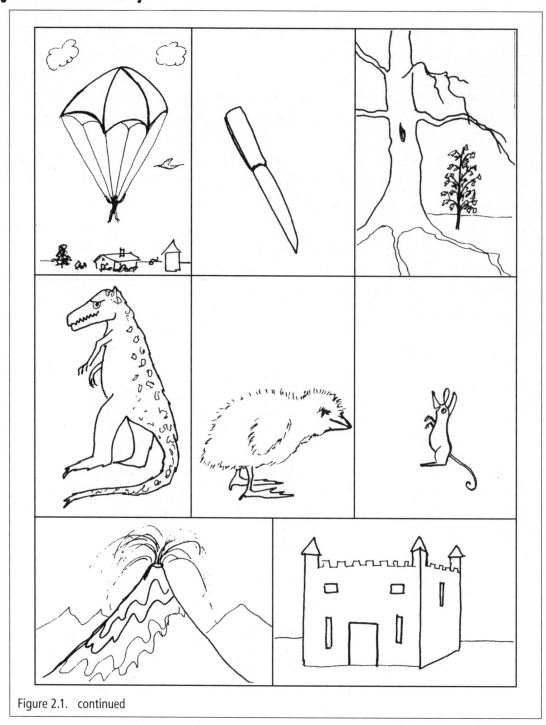

Figure 2.1. continued

The DAS assessment includes three rating scales that range from strongly negative (scored 1 point) to strongly positive (scored 5 points). The first two scales assess emotional content and self-image in response to the drawing task; the third scale is provided for response drawings that suggest humorous intent.

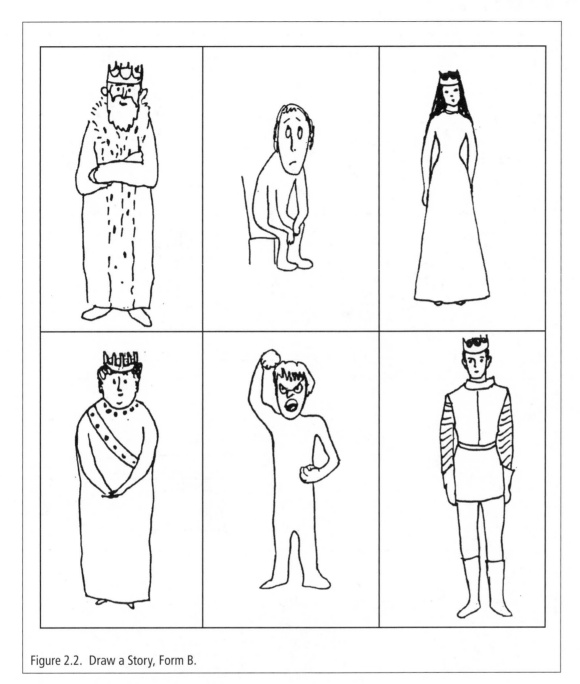

Figure 2.2. Draw a Story, Form B.

## The Scale for Assessing Emotional Content

The score of 1 point is used to identify strongly negative fantasies, such as solitary subjects in mortal danger or life-threatening relationships. The score of 5 points is used to identify strongly positive fantasies, such as successful solitary subjects or caring relationships. Moderately negative fantasies, such as unfortunate subjects and stressful relationships, score 2 points. Moderately positive fantasies, such as fortunate subjects and friendly relationships, score 4 points. Ambiguous or ambivalent subjects

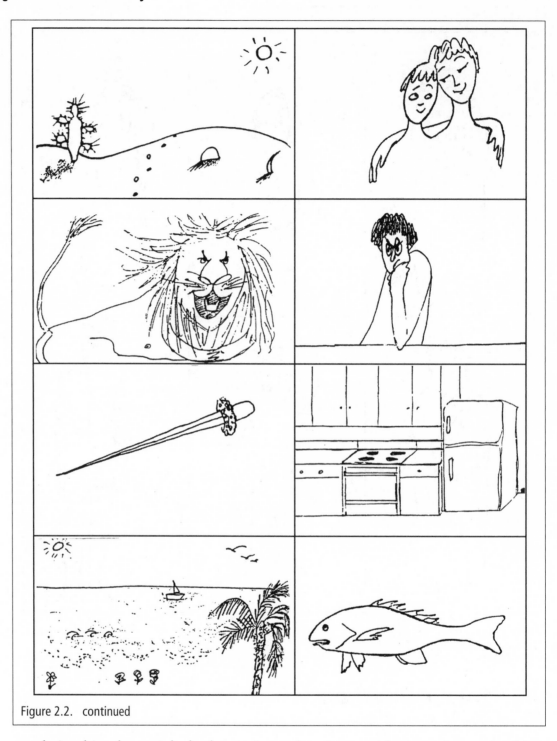

Figure 2.2. continued

or relationships that may be both negative and positive, neither negative nor positive, or else unclear, score 3 points.

The 3-point scale has been made more precise by adding scores of 2.5 and 3.5 points to identify ambiguous or ambivalent responses with hopeless or hopeful outcomes.

| Table 2.1 Scale for Assessing Emotional Content |
| --- |

___1 point: strongly negative emotional content; for example:

    Solitary subjects who appear sad, helpless, isolated, suicidal, dead, or in mortal danger

    Relationships that appear life threatening or lethal

___2 points: moderately negative emotional content; for example:

    Solitary subjects that appear frightened, angry, frustrated, dissatisfied, worried, destructive, or unfortunate

    Relationships that appear stressful, hostile, destructive, or unpleasant

___2.5 points: ambiguous or ambivalent emotional content suggesting unpleasant or unfortunate outcomes

___3 points: ambiguous or ambivalent emotional content; for example, both negative and positive, neither negative nor positive, unemotional, or unclear

___3.5 points: ambiguous or ambivalent emotional content suggesting hopeful, pleasant, or fortunate outcomes

___4 points: moderately positive emotional content; for example:

    Solitary subjects who appear fortunate but passive

    Relationships that appear friendly or positive

___5 points: strongly positive emotional content; for example:

    Solitary subjects who appear happy, effective, or to be achieving goals

    Relationships that are caring or loving

© 2007 Rawley Silver. Reprinted with permission for personal use only.

## The Scale for Assessing Self-Image

The aim of this scale is to identify subjects that may represent the person who responded to the drawing task. A response drawing that suggests the respondent identifies with a subject portrayed as sad, helpless, isolated, suicidal, or in mortal danger receives the lowest score of 1 point. A response that suggests the respondent identifies with a subject portrayed as happy, loved, admirable, powerful, intimidating, destructive, or achieving goals receives the highest score, 5 points. Ambiguous, ambivalent, or unemotional self-images score 3 points. Responses that suggest negative outcomes score 2.5 points; positive outcomes, 3.5 points. Moderately negative (frightened, frustrated, or unfortunate) self-images and moderately positive (fortunate but passive) self-images score 2 and 4 points, respectively.

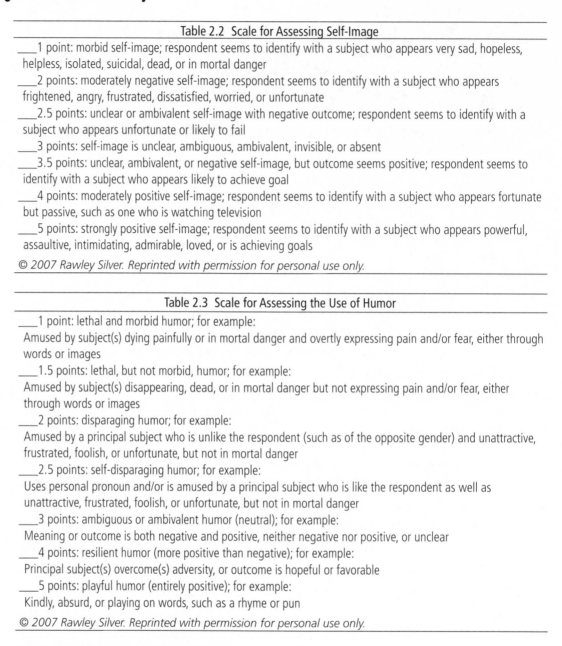

| Table 2.2  Scale for Assessing Self-Image |
|---|
| ____1 point: morbid self-image; respondent seems to identify with a subject who appears very sad, hopeless, helpless, isolated, suicidal, dead, or in mortal danger |
| ____2 points: moderately negative self-image; respondent seems to identify with a subject who appears frightened, angry, frustrated, dissatisfied, worried, or unfortunate |
| ____2.5 points: unclear or ambivalent self-image with negative outcome; respondent seems to identify with a subject who appears unfortunate or likely to fail |
| ____3 points: self-image is unclear, ambiguous, ambivalent, invisible, or absent |
| ____3.5 points: unclear, ambivalent, or negative self-image, but outcome seems positive; respondent seems to identify with a subject who appears likely to achieve goal |
| ____4 points: moderately positive self-image; respondent seems to identify with a subject who appears fortunate but passive, such as one who is watching television |
| ____5 points: strongly positive self-image; respondent seems to identify with a subject who appears powerful, assaultive, intimidating, admirable, loved, or is achieving goals |
| © 2007 Rawley Silver. Reprinted with permission for personal use only. |

| Table 2.3  Scale for Assessing the Use of Humor |
|---|
| ____1 point: lethal and morbid humor; for example: |
| Amused by subject(s) dying painfully or in mortal danger and overtly expressing pain and/or fear, either through words or images |
| ____1.5 points: lethal, but not morbid, humor; for example: |
| Amused by subject(s) disappearing, dead, or in mortal danger but not expressing pain and/or fear, either through words or images |
| ____2 points: disparaging humor; for example: |
| Amused by a principal subject who is unlike the respondent (such as of the opposite gender) and unattractive, frustrated, foolish, or unfortunate, but not in mortal danger |
| ____2.5 points: self-disparaging humor; for example: |
| Uses personal pronoun and/or is amused by a principal subject who is like the respondent as well as unattractive, frustrated, foolish, or unfortunate, but not in mortal danger |
| ____3 points: ambiguous or ambivalent humor (neutral); for example: |
| Meaning or outcome is both negative and positive, neither negative nor positive, or unclear |
| ____4 points: resilient humor (more positive than negative); for example: |
| Principal subject(s) overcome(s) adversity, or outcome is hopeful or favorable |
| ____5 points: playful humor (entirely positive); for example: |
| Kindly, absurd, or playing on words, such as a rhyme or pun |
| © 2007 Rawley Silver. Reprinted with permission for personal use only. |

## The Scale for Assessing the Use of Humor

Humorous responses that depict death or annihilation generally appear in two forms. The most negative seems morbid as well as lethal, scoring 1 point. It suggests that fantasizing about victims who are frightened or in pain, but die nevertheless, amuses the respondent. Lethal, but not morbid, humor—"gallows humor"—scores 1.5 points. It seems to laugh at death or annihilation, and tends to dispatch its victims without pain or grisly details, or out of sight. Disparaging humor, a response that shows ridiculed but unharmed subjects, also appears in two forms. The first, scored 2 points, makes fun of someone else's misfortunes. The second, self-disparaging humor, scoring 2.5 points, ridicules subjects who resemble the respondent. Responses that seem ambivalent, unemotional, or unclear score 3 points. Drawings about victims who joke about their fears or frustrations, that show resilient humor, score 4 points. Humor that seems motivated by high spirits and goodwill, with absurd subjects, witty titles, and little if any emotional involvement, scores 5 points.

**Drawing**

Story:_____

_____

_____

_____

_____

Please fill in the blanks below:

First name ____ Sex____ Age ____ Location (state): _____Date:_____

Just now I'm feeling ____very happy ____O.K. ____angry ____frightened ____sad

Figure 2.3. DAS Drawing Page.

## Examples of Scored Responses to the DAS Task

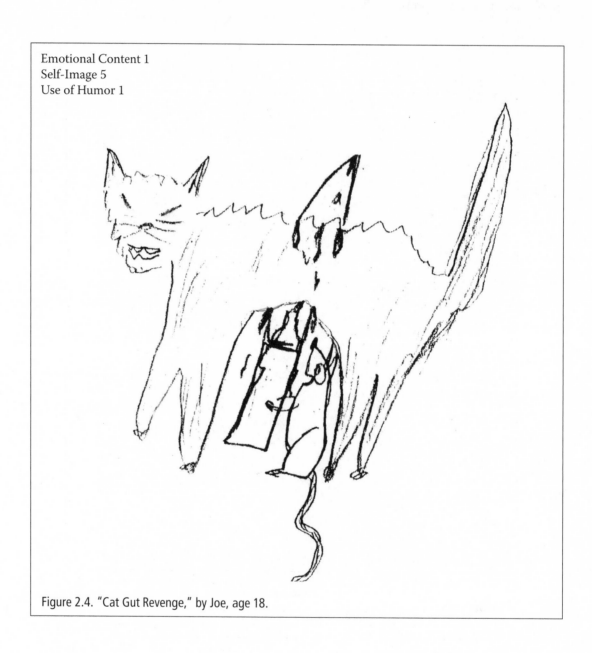

Emotional Content 1
Self-Image 5
Use of Humor 1

Figure 2.4. "Cat Gut Revenge," by Joe, age 18.

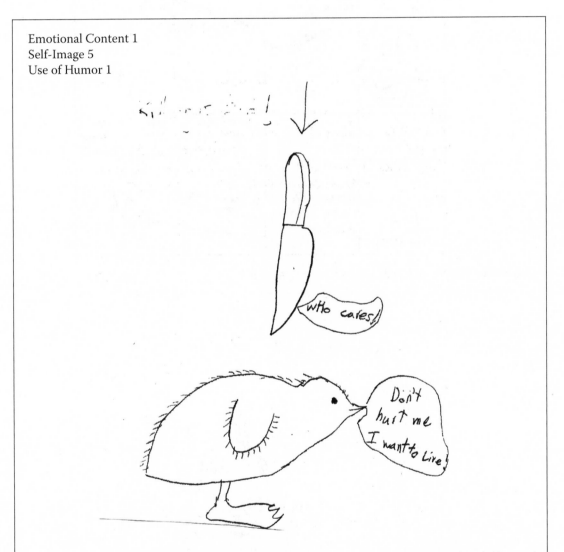

Emotional Content 1
Self-Image 5
Use of Humor 1

Figure 2.5. "Don't Hurt Me, I Want to Live. Who Cares," by Gus, age 12. Gus wrote, then half erased, "Killing is bad" at the top of the drawing.

Emotional Content 1
Self-Image 5
Use of Humor 1

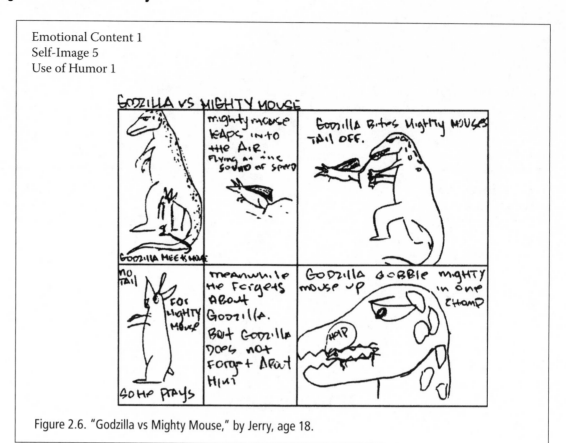

Figure 2.6. "Godzilla vs Mighty Mouse," by Jerry, age 18.

Emotional Content 1
Self-Image 3
Use of Humor 1.5

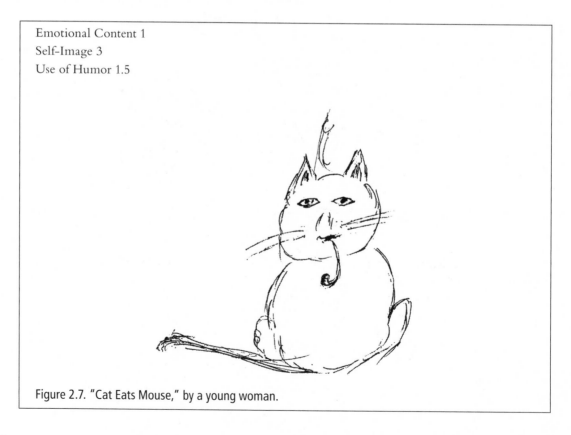

Figure 2.7. "Cat Eats Mouse," by a young woman.

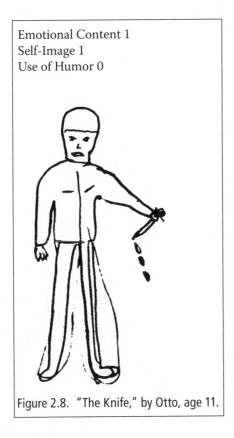

Emotional Content 1
Self-Image 1
Use of Humor 0

Figure 2.8. "The Knife," by Otto, age 11.

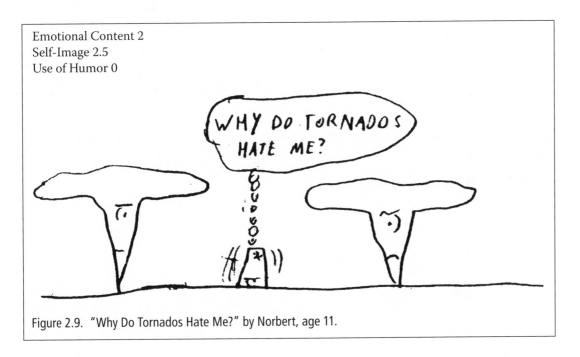

Emotional Content 2
Self-Image 2.5
Use of Humor 0

Figure 2.9. "Why Do Tornados Hate Me?" by Norbert, age 11.

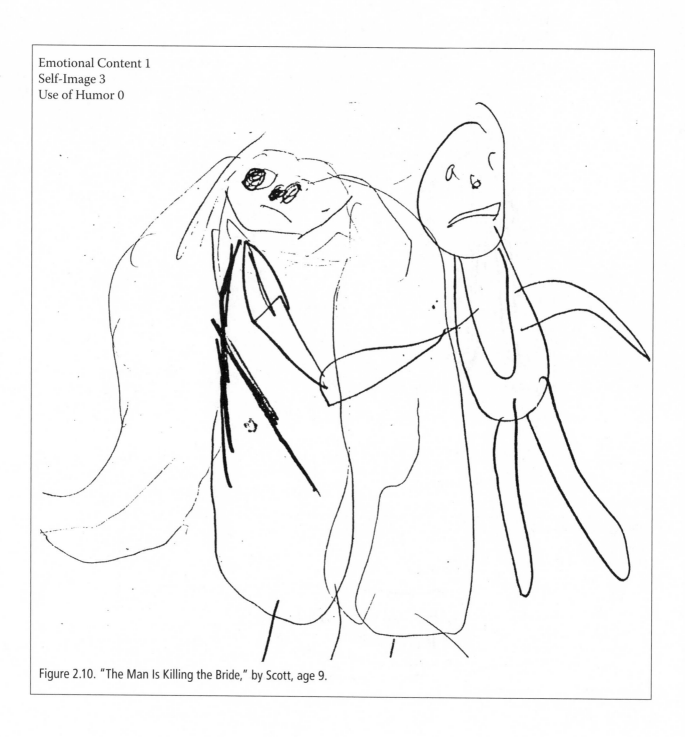

Emotional Content 1
Self-Image 3
Use of Humor 0

Figure 2.10. "The Man Is Killing the Bride," by Scott, age 9.

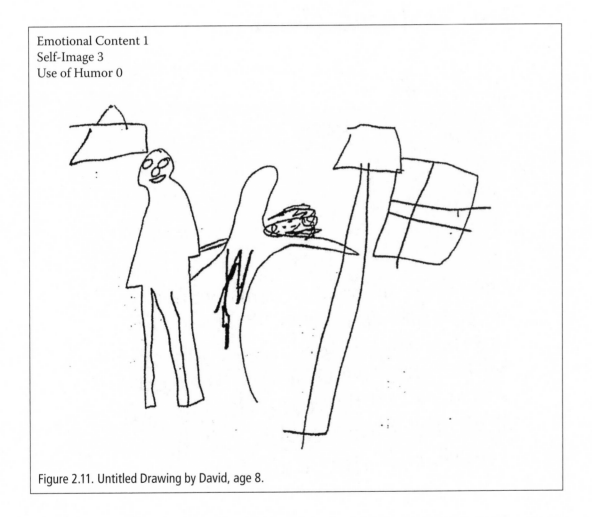

Emotional Content 1
Self-Image 3
Use of Humor 0

Figure 2.11. Untitled Drawing by David, age 8.

Emotional Content 1
Self-Image 1
Use of Humor 0

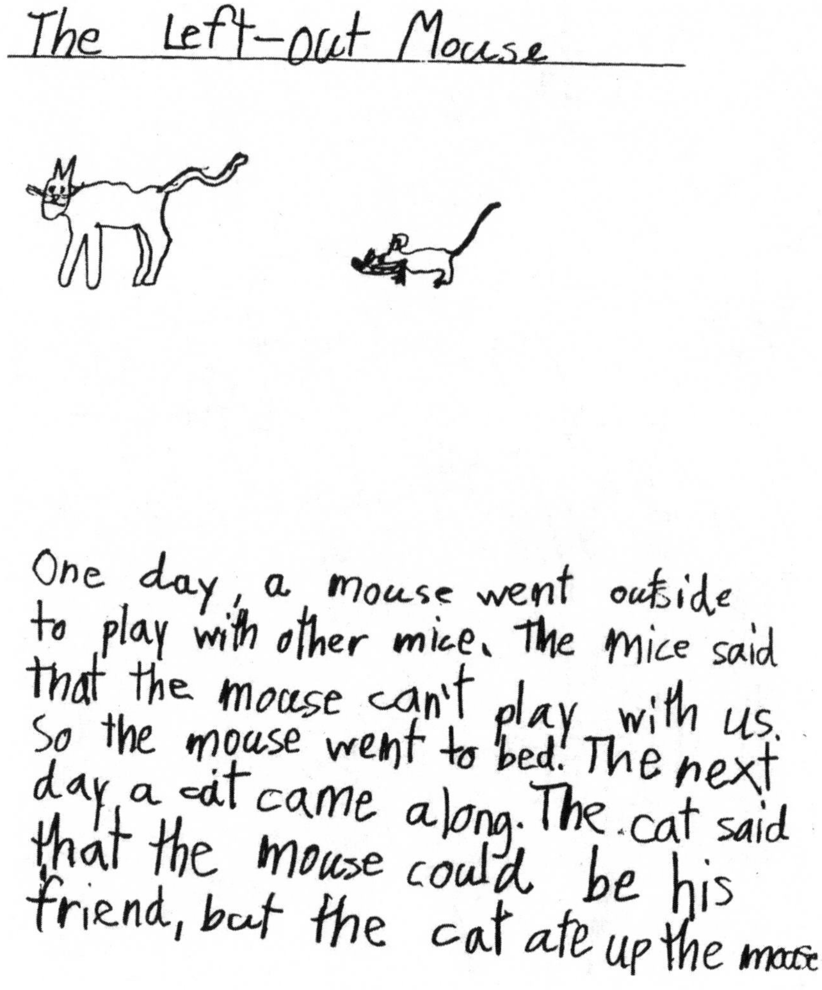

The Left-out Mouse

One day, a mouse went outside
to play with other mice. The mice said
that the mouse can't play with us.
So the mouse went to bed. The next
day a cat came along. The cat said
that the mouse could be his
friend, but the cat ate up the mouse

Figure 2.12. "The Left-Out Mouse," by Gerald, age 8.

Emotional Content 2
Self-Image 5
Use of Humor 2

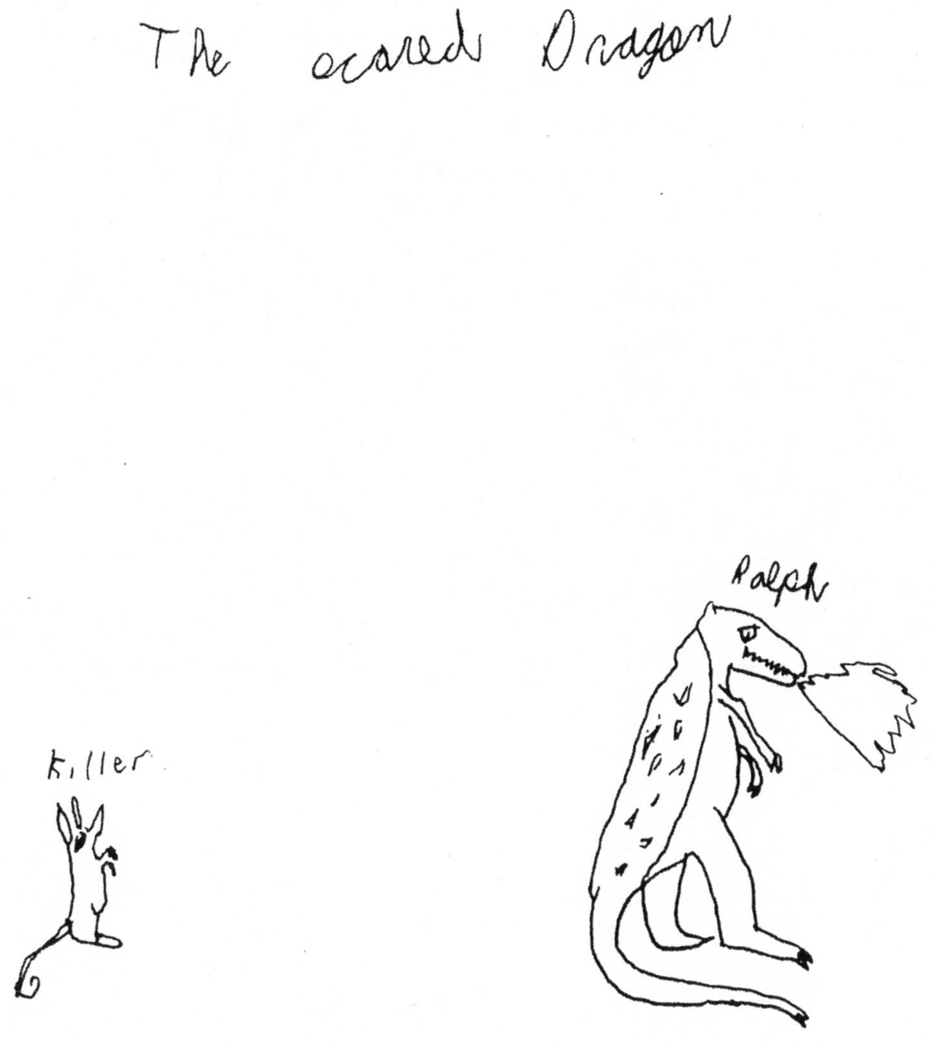

The scared Dragon

Ralph

killer

Figure 2.13. "There Was a Dragon Named Ralph Who Was Scared of a Killer Mouse," by Ezra, age 16.

Emotional Content 2
Self-Image 2
Use of Humor 2.5

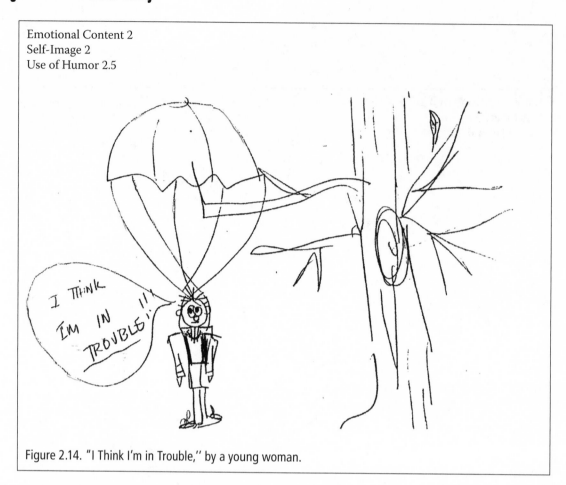

Figure 2.14. "I Think I'm in Trouble," by a young woman.

Emotional Content 2.5
Self-Image 5
Use of Humor 1.5

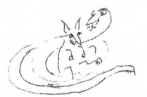

Figure 2.15. "The Snake and the Mouse," by a senior man (good for the snake, bad for the mouse).

Emotional Content 4
Self-Image 4
Use of Humor 5

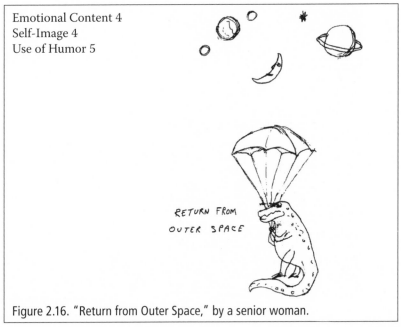

Figure 2.16. "Return from Outer Space," by a senior woman.

Emotional Content 3
Self-Image 3
Use of Humor 5

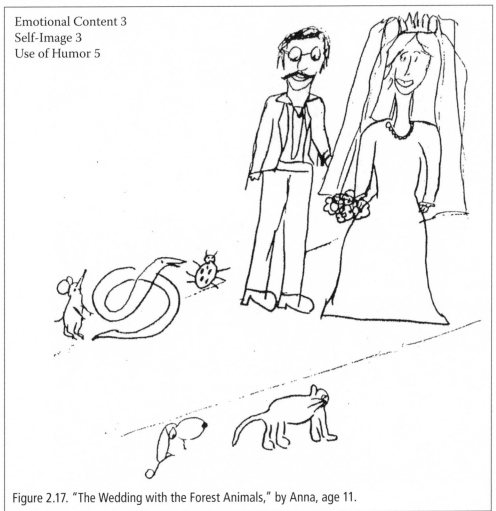

Figure 2.17. "The Wedding with the Forest Animals," by Anna, age 11.

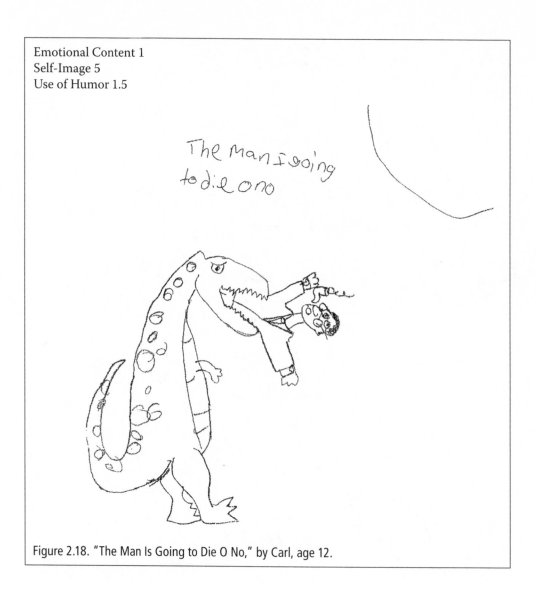

Emotional Content 1
Self-Image 5
Use of Humor 1.5

The Man I going to die o no

Figure 2.18. "The Man Is Going to Die O No," by Carl, age 12.

# Chapter 3

# Reliability, Validity, and Depression

◇   ◇   ◇

To have reliability and validity, the Draw a Story (DAS) assessment should provide criteria that accord with diagnostic criteria in the literature. In addition, it should show consistency among scorers, as well as retest consistency over periods of time, and its premises should be supported by quantified evidence. This chapter begins with a question, suggests answers, presents diagnostic criteria, and then proceeds to studies of reliability and validity.

How is it that we can we look at drawings made by strangers and understand how they feel about themselves and others? Neuroscientists have proposed that the underlying mechanism is the brain's mirror neuron system; the brain is able to link "I do and I feel" with "he does and he feels," as discussed in chapter 1. Tinen (1990a) has suggested that the ability to perceive and interpret nonverbal messages expressed through art forms is based on unconscious mimicry, and that mimicry underlies empathy and aesthetic sensibility.

## Diagnostic Criteria

Responses to the drawing task with strongly negative emotional content and self-image are scored 1 point, based on the symptoms of depression cited by Beck, Rush,

Shaw, and Emory (1979), McKnew, Cytryn, and Yahries (1983), Pfeffer (1986), and Shaffer and Fisher (1981), as discussed in chapter 2. In addition, the diagnostic criteria cited in *Diagnostic Criteria from DSM-IV* (American Psychiatric Association, 1994) notes feelings of hopelessness and low self-esteem.

Gantt and Tabone (1998) have noted that drawings by depressed patients have distinct patterns and seem closer to normal controls than drawings by those with organic mental disorders or schizophrenia. They found no significant differences between drawings by patients who were depressed and those of control group patients in problem solving, logic, integration, and realism. They differed from drawings by other psychiatric patients, however, by showing greater use of logic and better problem-solving skills, and they differed from patients with organic mental disorders by showing a significant increase in energy, integration, logic, and ability to solve problems.

Wadeson (1980) has emphasized the formal attributes of drawings, such as the use of color or space. She asked depressed patients to make spontaneous drawings with colored chalks, and found that their drawings showed more empty space than did the drawings of nondepressed individuals, showing less color, less effort, and either less affect or more depressive affect, such as that of harming others.

The DAS assessment evaluates the content of responses to the drawing task rather than their formal attributes. Originally published in 1988, revised editions were published in 1993, 1996, and 2002.

Practitioners in various parts of the country volunteered to administer the DAS assessment to 1,028 children, adolescents, and adults. They included 446 subjects with no known impairments residing in Florida, Kansas, New Jersey, New York, Minnesota, Missouri, and Ohio; and 449 emotionally disturbed, clinically depressed, delinquent, or learning-disabled subjects in Arizona, California, Florida, Georgia, New Jersey, New York, Maine, Minnesota, Montana, Oregon, and Pennsylvania. Most of these test booklet responses were donated to the archives of the American Art Therapy Association.

## The Scale for Assessing Emotional Content

To determine scorer reliability, three registered art therapists scored 20 unidentified responses to DAS Form A (Silver, 1993a, 2002). The responses were chosen at random from five clinical and nonclinical groups of children and adolescents. Before scoring, the judges met for about an hour to discuss scoring procedures, then scored the responses blindly and independently. Madeline Altabe, PhD, then performed the statistical analyses. She found the correlations among scores highly significant, at the .001 level of probability. Between judges A and B, the correlation coefficient was .806 (df = 18, $p < .001$); between judges A and C, .749 (df = 18, $p < .001$) and between judges B and C, .816 (df = 18, $p < .001$).

To determine retest reliability, 24 third-graders were presented with the Form A task on two occasions (Silver, 1993a, 2002). Twelve of these presumably normal children responded with strongly or moderately negative fantasies. When they were retested after an interval of approximately one month, seven received the same scores, three had higher scores, and two had lower scores (from 2 points to 1 point). When 12 other children were retested after an interval of approximately two years, 11 received the same scores they had received previously (Silver, 1993a).

Subsequently, three registered art therapists on two occasions presented the Form A set of stimulus drawings to children and adults who responded (Silver, 1993a, 2002). One therapist presented the task twice after a one-week interval to eight children with emotional disturbances in a New Jersey public elementary school. The second presented the task without a time interval to six adolescents with emotional disturbances, ages 14 to 18, in a summer art therapy program in Florida. The third presented it to 17 men and women in Florida who volunteered to participate anonymously. Significant correlations were found between the first and second responses of the 31 subjects (.70262, $p < 0.000$). Correlation for the 8 children was .93277 ($p < 0.000$), and for the adolescents and adults combined, .45095 ($p < .05$).

In addition, the retest and scorer reliability of DAS Form B was examined (Silver, 1993c). In this study, 33 children, adolescents, and adults responded twice. They included normal subjects as well as those who had been diagnosed previously as depressed or emotionally disturbed, or else had attention deficit disorders or learning disabilities.

Two judges independently scored the responses, which were identified only by number. They scored first and second drawings on different days. To determine the degree of their agreement in assigning scores, separate interscorer correlations were calculated for the first 33 responses marked A, the 33 second responses marked B, and the combined 66 A/B responses. Interscorer correlations were significant. The correlation for A scores was .83943 ($p < 0.000$); for B scores, .74054; and for combined A and B scores, .80806 ($p < 0.000$).

Based on these findings, the scale for assessing emotional content seems reliable. The findings also suggest a link between depressive illness and strongly negative responses. Although strongly negative responses do not necessarily indicate depression and, conversely, positive responses do not exclude depression, they suggest that a child or adolescent scoring 1 point may be at risk for depression.

The findings also indicated that negative feelings persisted over time, suggesting that they reflected characteristic attitudes rather than passing moods. These observations were supported in the studies of depression that are reviewed in chapter 5.

## The Scale for Assessing Self-Image

Studies of the reliability and validity of the self-image scale began with a study published in 1992. It asked whether children tend to draw fantasies about people the same gender as themselves when responding to the drawing task (Silver, 1992). In search of answers, the responses of 261 children were reviewed, comparing their genders with the genders of the subjects they drew. The children included 145 boys and 116 girls: second-, third-, and fourth-graders, ages 7 to 10, in eight public elementary schools in urban and suburban neighborhoods in four states and in Canada.

Results indicated that the children drew pictures about people of the same genders as themselves to a highly significant degree, and gender differences were significant at the .001 level of probability.

A second study examined attitudes toward self and others, as well as same-gender subjects, and expanded the number of participants to 531 adults, adolescents, and children. They included 257 males and 274 females in five age groups: 7 to 10, 13 to 16, 17 to 19, 20 to 50, and 65 or older (Silver, 1993b). Their responses were divided into two groups—drawings about solitary subjects, and drawings about relationships among subjects—and then examined for differences and similarities.

Most respondents drew fantasies about subjects of the same gender as themselves to a highly significant degree. Using two-by-two chi-square analysis, the findings indicated that respondents who drew human subjects chose same-gender subjects to a degree significant at the .001 level of probability ($\chi^2 = 145.839$; $p < .001$; $0 = .657$).

The tendency to choose same-gender subjects peaked in childhood and reached its lowest level among young adults. Among senior adults, however, gender differences emerged. Although the decline continued among older women, it reversed among older men, most of whom chose male subjects.

In addition, proportionally more women and girls expressed positive attitudes toward solitary subjects, but their drawings about relationships were both positive and negative. These findings were also significant at the .001 level of probability ($\chi^2 = 25.32$; $p < .001$).

On the other hand, males showed higher frequency than females in drawings about assaultive relationships ($\chi^2[1] = 9.38$; $p < .01$). However, gender and age differences interacted, resulting in significant age variability for females, but not males. That is, female fantasies about assaults change with age. Proportionally more of the older women drew fantasies about assaulting others than any other age or gender group, whereas male fantasies about assaults remained stable.

In drawing about caring relationships, the converse age and gender interaction was found. Males showed significant age variability, whereas females had similar frequency across age groups. In addition, proportionally more of the young men fantasized about caring relationships than any other age or gender group.

In drawings about stressful relationships, scored 2 points, more of the senior men drew fantasies about stressful relationships than any other age or gender group, whereas little difference between genders emerged.

## Identifying Self-Images without Meeting the Adolescents Who Drew Them

It is often claimed that in order to identify self-images in a drawing, practitioners must discuss the drawing with the person who drew it in order to avoid projecting the practitioners' own feelings into the drawing.

To investigate the claim, we asked whether self-images can be identified without meeting and talking with the person who drew it, and whether art therapists and social workers agree when identifying self-images (Silver & Ellison, 1995). The term *self-image* is defined as one or more characters in a drawing that represent the person who drew it, intentionally or unintentionally.

Ellison, a registered art therapist who worked with adolescents in a residential detention facility in California, presented the DAS Form B task to 53 youths, ages 13 to 18, and then discussed their drawings with them individually. She also asked them to identify characters in their drawings that might represent themselves. She then sent only the drawings to me in New York. Altabe evaluated the three sets of evaluations, using the level of agreement between the 39 adolescents, Ellison, and myself, as an index of the validity of the self-image measure.

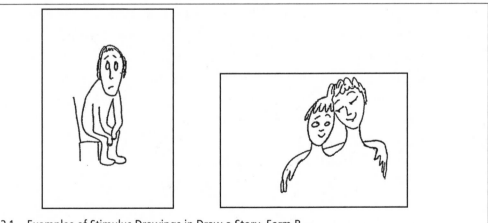

Figure 3.1.   Examples of Stimulus Drawings in Draw a Story, Form B.

In addition, three other art therapists and five social workers rated self-images in 10 of the 53 response drawings, selected at random. Agreements among the respondents, art therapists, and social workers were also analyzed.

Of the 53 adolescents, 39 identified characters in their drawings as themselves. Ellison, who knew their histories and conducted the interviews, accurately matched 77% of the adolescents in identifying their self-images. Judging blindly, I matched 72%. Between us the agreement was 94.3%, suggesting interscorer reliability.

The average agreement among the five social workers was 54%; among the five art therapists, 78%; and among the subgroup of registered art therapists, 93%. Overall, the 10 judges agreed 61% of the time. There was some inconsistency in raters' responses. Specifically, not all raters rated each individual, and some raters gave an individual more than one rating.

In addition, the level of agreement among the 39 adolescents and the two registered art therapists was examined. Approximately three of four respondents (74.4%) agreed with the art therapists. Ellison agreed with two respondents who disagreed with Silver, suggesting that the absence of discussion caused me to incorrectly judge two of the 39 responses.

Although five respondents disagreed with both Ellison and me about the identity of their self-images, Ellison and I agreed with each other. For example, figure 3.2 is the response by Chris, age 16, who had chosen two stimulus drawings, the dejected person sitting in a chair and the couple with arms entwined.

> "The man hear is very sad because he got an F on his spelling test. He is really depressed because he tried his hardest and failed. He doesn't have answers to a better grade. The other people in this story are very happy. They both got As in their spelling test. They got good grades by helping each other. The other person who got an F was mad that he had the chance to be part of these peoples group but he decided to do it alone."

Chris was performing at the fourth-grade level in spelling but at the seventh- and eighth-grade levels in reading and math. When Ellison asked him how he imagined the characters in his drawing might feel, he described the dejected person as "sad and depressed" and the couple as "happy." When she asked how he would feel if he were in the picture, he replied that he "would be part of the group."

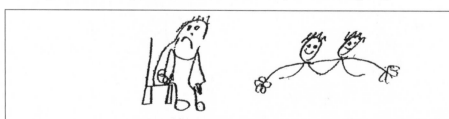

Figure 3.2. "The Man Hear Is Very Sad Because He Got an F on His Spelling Test," by Chris, age 16.

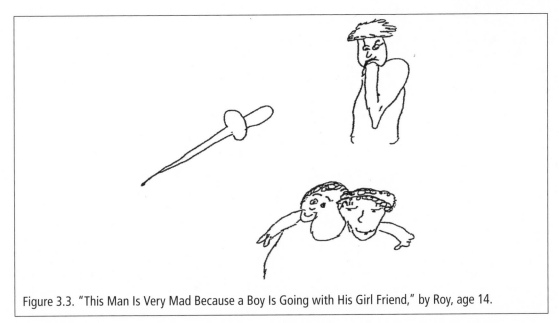

Figure 3.3. "This Man Is Very Mad Because a Boy Is Going with His Girl Friend," by Roy, age 14.

Figure 3.3 is the response by Roy, age 14, who chose three stimulus drawings—the angry person, the sword, and the loving couple—and wrote, "The man is very mad because a boy is going with his girl friend, the two [*sic*] couple don't know her boyfriend is watching, so he's going to grab the knife and kill both of them."

Asked how he imagined his characters might feel, Roy said the man was very angry, the boy and girl were happy, and if he were in the picture, he would be the boy with the girl: "I'm the good guy. I couldn't kill nobody."

Ellison and I disagreed with both Chris and with Roy, but agreed with each other that the sad man represented Chris and the angry man represented Roy.

Both social work and art therapy require training in psychotherapy, and both require master's degrees. Nevertheless, as judges, the art therapists and social workers tended to perceive the drawings differently.

For example, Larry, age 13, chose stimulus drawings of the king, queen, and kitchen; he then drew Figure 3.4, adding, "This is a piture [*sic*] of my Mom and Dad in the kitchen cook me a meal on a Sunday morning."

The three registered art therapists indicated that Larry had omitted himself from his drawing. The seven other judges identified the man, or both the man and woman, as Larry's self-image. When Larry was asked how he would feel if he were in the picture, he replied, "I'm in the other room at a table, waiting for breakfast."

How can the differences in scoring be explained? Social workers are mental health professionals, and art therapists tend to be artists with training in psychotherapy. It may be that mirror neuron mechanisms described in chapter 1 were more activated in the brains of the art therapists because of their experiences as artists, stimulating

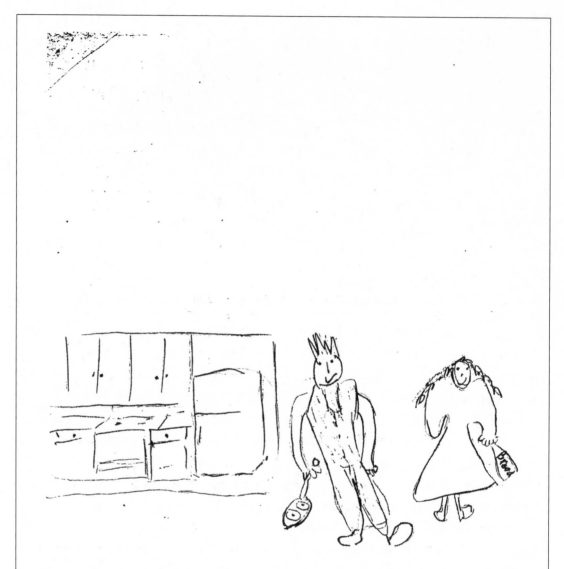

Figure 3.4. "This Is a Piture of My Mom and Dad in the Kitchen Cook Me a Meal on a Sunday Morning," by Larry, age 12.

their empathy circuits more intensely, and enabling them to internalize more readily the feelings expressed in drawings by others.

To replicate the study with a larger sample of mental health professionals, 29 emotional health counselors with master's degrees evaluated the same 10 response drawings, using the same scoring form. Their experiences as school counselors in Florida averaged 19.09 years. Five judges were eliminated either because they wrote "yes" instead of identifying the self-images or because they did not provide information about their educational backgrounds.

Like the art therapists in the previous study, 22 of the 24 judges (92%) disagreed with Chris, who drew figure 3.2, and agreed with each other, identifying the sad man as his self-image, and agreeing that he felt unfortunate. In addition, 23 of the 24 judges indicated that Chris was not aggressive.

Similarly, 22 of the 24 judges disagreed with Roy, who drew figure 3.3, and identified the angry man in his drawing as Roy's self-image. Twenty-two also checked "unfortunate," and 21 "aggressive."

However, in judging figure 3.4, Larry's drawing of his mother and father in the kitchen, only 10 (42%) found no self-image; 15 (63%) indicated more than one, 9 (38%) indicated that he identified with his parents, and 5 (21%) indicated that the drawing was unclear.

The agreement among the emotional health counselors, like the agreement among the art therapists in the previous study, suggests that most perceived covert fears and wishes, even though they had not met Roy and Chris and knew nothing of their histories. The different levels of agreement suggest that some may be unable to recognize self-images in drawings, whereas others are able to do so without discussion if need be, perhaps because they have developed the mirror neurons being tracked by neuroscientists using magnetic resonance imaging, or MRI, scans.

I believe that what children or adults say about their drawings is no less important than the drawings themselves. That is why the drawing page of the DAS assessment includes the questions on the bottom of the page. Even though hospitalized depressed patients may have checked "very happy," their words provide useful clues and openings for discussion. But there are times when it is impossible to discuss response drawings with the individuals who drew them, and decisions must be made. The study with Ellison was a search for answers to the question whether images can be identified without discussion if need be.

## The Validity and Reliability of the Emotional Content and Self-Image Scales

The DAS scales are essentially the same as the Silver Drawing Test (SDT) scales for assessing emotional content and self-image, and they share 7 of their 15 stimulus drawings. Studies found that DAS and the SDT assess the same constructs, lending evidence to the validity of scores across test formats (Silver, 2002, pp. 224–230). A study of scorer reliability found strong reliability for the emotional content scale (0.94) and moderate reliability for the self-image scale (0.74) (Silver, 1996c, 2002). The present scales have changed some phrasing and added scores of 2.5 and 3.5 points for ambiguous or ambivalent responses that suggest unfortunate or fortunate outcomes, respectively.

To determine whether the changes might affect the scales' reliability, four art therapists who had received both registration and board certification from the American Art Therapy Association scored responses to the drawing task by ten children and adolescents, ages 8 to 17, six boys and four girls. The judges had no special training but had been using the drawing task for several years. They skipped the customary practice session; that is, they did not discuss a preliminary set of stimulus drawings until they agreed on the meaning of each score. Instead, I sent the same set of ten response drawings to each judge. They scored the responses independently and blindly, knowing only the titles of the drawings and the age and gender of each respondent, then mailed their scores directly to Madeline Altabe, PhD, for statistical analysis.

Interscorer agreement on the self-image and emotional content scales was calculated as 80% and 82.5%, respectively. This finding represents good agreement across raters in evaluating response drawings by children and adolescents.

## The Scale for Assessing the Use of Humor

To find humorous responses to the drawing task, we reviewed 849 responses to the Drawing from Imagination task of the DAS and SDT assessments, finding 142 drawings (16%) that suggested humorous intent (Silver, 2001, 2002, 2003).

To determine the reliability of the Scale for Assessing the Use of Humor (see table 2.3 in chapter 2), three judges scored 12 humorous responses from children, adolescents, young adults, and senior adults. The judges included two registered art therapists with board certification and an art therapist who had recently received the master's degree. Because they lived in different states, they discussed the scores via telephone and e-mail after scoring a preliminary set of 15 humorous responses. When they felt they had come to agreement in scoring the responses, they scored a second set of 12 humorous responses blindly, independently, and without discussion, and then mailed their scores directly to Brooke Butler, PhD, for statistical analysis. Butler found a reliability coefficient of 0.861, which exceeds the minimum level of acceptability (0.80), and suggests that the humor scale is reliable.

## Studies of Depression

A first study asked whether strongly negative responses to the DAS task were associated with clinical depression (Silver, 1988a). A few children, adolescents, and adults had responded to the SDT Drawing from Imagination task with fantasies about suicide, and more than a few drew fantasies about death, dying, or hopeless situations. Were they depressed? In search of answers, I selected a new set of 14 stimulus drawings that later became Form A of the DAS assessment. Nineteen art therapists, teachers, and school counselors volunteered to administer the task to 248 children and adolescents who ranged in age from 8 to 21 and resided in Arizona, Montana,

New Jersey, New York, Oregon, and Pennsylvania. The subjects included 21 who had been diagnosed previously as clinically depressed, 61 who had emotional disturbances with nondepressive psychopathology, 31 with learning disabilities, 111 who presumably were not depressed, and 24 who responded to the drawing task on two occasions.

Approximately 56% of the depressed subjects responded to the drawing task with strongly negative fantasies scoring 1 point, compared with 11% of the unimpaired group, 21% of those with emotional disturbances, and 32% of those with learning disabilities.

To determine whether the differences were significant, a chi-square analysis found that significantly more depressed than nondepressed subjects scored 1 point (27.63, $p < .001$). The proportion of depressed subjects scoring 1 point also was significantly greater than the proportion of emotionally disturbed subjects scoring 1 point (10.54, $p < .01$) but not significantly greater than the proportion of subjects with learning disabilities (3.269, $p < .05$). In addition, the study found that most of the 24 children who responded to the drawing task on two occasions received the same scores. The findings suggested that strongly negative responses scoring 1 point are associated with adolescent or childhood depression, and that the drawing task might be useful as a first step in identifying depressed children and adolescents.

Building on these findings, a second study increased the number of subjects to 350 children and adolescents, and asked whether strongly negative responses to the DAS task were associated with clinical depression (Silver, 1988b). Twenty-four art therapists, teachers, and school counselors volunteered their assistance.

The subjects included 35 children or adolescents with depression, 15 adults with depression, 117 presumably normal children and adolescents, 74 children and adolescents with emotional disturbances and nondepressive psychopathology, 64 adolescents with learning disabilities, 18 children and adolescents with hearing impairments, and 27 older adults. Their responses also were evaluated on a scale ranging from strongly negative to strongly positive themes.

Approximately 63% of the children and adolescents with depression responded with strongly negative themes, scoring 1 point, whereas approximately 10% of the nondepressed children and adolescents scored 1 point, as shown in figure 3.5, DAS Responses from Depressed and Nondepressed Subjects.

To determine whether the differences were significant, a chi-square analysis was conducted. The proportion of children and adolescents with depression scoring 1 point was significantly greater than the proportion of any other group scoring 1 point: compared with the presumably normal children and adolescents, the chi square was 43.2 ($p < .0005$); compared with that of people who had emotional

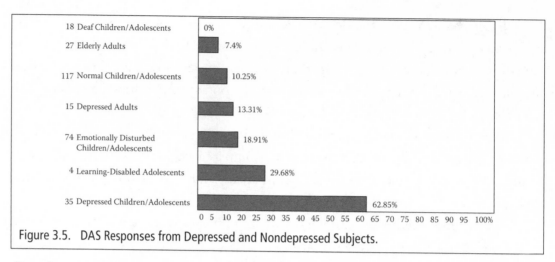

Figure 3.5. DAS Responses from Depressed and Nondepressed Subjects.

disturbances, 20.6 ($p < .0005$); compared with that of subjects who had learning disabilities, 11.1 ($p < .001$); compared with that of subjects who had hearing impairments, 19.5 ($p < .0005$); compared with that of older persons, 20.0 ($p < .0005$); and compared with the chi square of adults with depression, 10.4 ($p < .005$).

These findings suggest that strongly negative responses to the DAS assessment are associated with adolescent or childhood depression. They also suggest that the DAS instrument could serve as a first step in identifying some, but not all, children and adolescents with depression. Although strongly negative responses did not necessarily indicate depression—and, conversely, positive responses did not exclude depression—the findings seem to indicate that a child or adolescent who responds with a strongly negative fantasy may be at risk, and that further examination by a mental health professional would be justified.

The findings about children and adolescents with depression did not apply to adults with depression. Only 2 of the 11 adults with depression scored 1 point, whereas 9 received the neutral score of 3 points (ambivalent, ambiguous, or unemotional).

Did this indicate that responses by depressed adults tend to be ambivalent, ambiguous, unemotional, or more guarded than responses by children and adolescents with depression? Were the adults being treated more successfully? Would a self-report or evaluation of the use of space or detail clarify the responses?

A third study examined age and gender differences in responses to the DAS task by 103 adults and adolescents with and without depression (Silver, 1993a). The depressed sample included 47 patients hospitalized for depression in Georgia (18 girls and women, ages 12 to 69; and 23 boys and men, ages 17 to 53). The nondepressed sample included university students in Florida and residents of a nursing home in Pennsylvania (34 women, ages 19 to 72; and 26 men, ages 20 to 77). The study also included a self-report and scales for assessing the use of space and detail.

Based on an analysis of variance for depression and the use of space and detail, no significant effects emerged for the depressed groups, no difference emerged in the use of space, and only gender differences emerged in the use of detail ($F$ [1,103] = 4.27; $p$ < .05). Females used significantly less detail (mean = 1.84) than males (mean = 2.31).

Findings of the three studies suggest that strongly negative responses to the DAS assessment are associated with childhood depression and may be associated with depression among adolescents and men. The association with adolescent depression is unclear, because the adolescent samples were combined with other samples in both studies. In the first study (Silver, 1988a), adolescents with depression were combined with children who had depression because the samples were too small for separate statistical analyses. For the same reason, the 1993 study combined the sample of 7 male adolescents with depression with the 15 men who had depression, and the 7 female adolescents with depression with the 18 women who had depression.

Although the men with depression responded with negative themes to a significant degree, the significance of their difference from nondepressed males was borderline.

The studies did not find that strongly negative responses to the DAS task were associated with depression in women. However, the question remains as to whether neutral responses are associated. The second study (Silver, 1998b) found that 9 of the adults with depression responded with neutral themes; the 1993 study found that the chi-square analysis was significant for the group with depression and that females with depression tended to produce drawings with neutral themes. This raises the question of whether depression among women is associated with ambivalent or ambiguous themes (comparatively few women drew pictures with unemotional themes).

When the two formal attributes of drawings were evaluated, the drawings of female respondents showed significantly fewer details than those of male respondents, but no difference was found between the drawings by subjects with depression and those by nondepressed subjects, either in the use of detail or in the use of space. Consequently, the scale for assessing space and detail was eliminated.

Because no significant difference was found between respondents with depression and nondepressed respondents, either in the use of detail or the use of space, scales for assessing space and detail were eliminated from the DAS assessment. The self-report, however, has been retained for reasons that will follow.

## The Self-Report and Masked Depression

The brief self-report below the written story asks respondents to check the appropriate empty space in the sentence, "Just now I'm feeling—very happy—O.K.—

angry—frightened—sad." Surprisingly, most examinees responded by checking "very happy" or "O.K.," even when they were hospitalized for clinical depression and drew pictures about sadness or death. The inconsistency suggested that they were in fact depressed, but that reticence, denial, the effects of antidepressant medication, or responding in the presence of others discouraged a thoughtful response. It also may be that drawings are less guarded than words; less vulnerable to denial than traditional, verbal self-reports; or less vulnerable to conscious deception and the desire to please. At any event, we found that even misleading self-reports were useful in follow-up discussions. Consequently, the self-report remains in the DAS assessment.

## Chapter 4

# Aggression and Depression

◇     ◇     ◇

**V**iolent behavior seems to be increasing and aggressive incidents occur frequently in schools, as was discussed in chapter 2. The number of seriously injured children nearly quadrupled from 1986 to 1993, and other children inflicted a substantial proportion of their injuries (Bok, 1998). Prevention of violence has become a priority in schools throughout the country.

In a study of responses by delinquent and nondelinquent adolescents to the Draw a Story (DAS) assessment, it was surprising to find that more boys in the nondelinquent group drew fantasies about assaultive relationships than boys in the delinquent group.

## Comparing Aggressive and Nonaggressive Groups

Three studies compared groups of students with histories of aggressive behavior and control groups of students with no histories of aggression. The first study examined DAS assessment responses from 138 delinquent and nondelinquent adolescents, ages 13 to 17 (Silver, 1996b). The delinquent group included 53 boys and 11 girls attending English classes in a residential treatment facility for incarcerated adolescents in California. The nondelinquent group included 29 boys and 45 girls attending English classes in four schools in Ohio, New York, and Florida. Their responses were divided into four groups—delinquency, gender, drawings about relationships, and drawings about solitary subjects—and then evaluated on the scales for assessing emotional content, self-image, and the use of humor (see chapter 2).

The first analysis evaluated whether gender or delinquency were related to self-image scores. No significant differences were found. The second analysis evaluated whether the proportions of drawings about solitary subjects or assaultive relationships differed depending on gender or delinquency. Significant gender differences emerged in both solitary and assaultive content: more boys than girls drew pictures about assaultive relationships (32% boys, 5% girls) and more girls than boys drew fantasies about solitary subjects (38% girls, 16% boys). Although the nondelinquent boys differed significantly from nondelinquent girls, no gender differences appeared in the delinquent groups.

Delinquency also made a difference in positive responses, scored 4 and 5 points. More than three times as many nondelinquent as delinquent adolescents drew fortunate solitary subjects (14% vs 4%). No delinquent girls, but 20% of the nondelinquent girls, drew fortunate solitary subjects. None of the delinquent girls expressed positive feelings toward their solitary subjects. These findings suggest that delinquent behavior, when followed by incarceration, dims or extinguishes wish-fulfilling fantasies and hopes for success.

A subsequent study asked whether responses to the Draw a Story assessment by aggressive children and adolescents have distinctive characteristics that can be quantified and scored, and whether there were significant differences between their scores and a control group of presumably nonaggressive students (Earwood, Fedorko, Holzman, Montanari, & Silver, 2004). Four art therapists in four schools presented the DAS Form A to 30 students they knew had histories of aggressive behavior and to 181 students with no histories of aggressive behavior who served as the control group.

The students, ages 8 to 19, were attending English or art classes in four public elementary or secondary schools in Florida and New Jersey. Two schools were in upper- to middle-class neighborhoods; the other two were in low- to middle-class neighborhoods. The aggressive group included 25 boys and 5 girls. Seven attended a school that does not have an art therapy program, whereas 23 attended three schools that do provide these programs. The parents of these students had given permission for them to participate in the study, and Brooke Butler, PhD, analyzed the findings using analyses of variance (ANOVA).

# Results

The aggressive group had lower, more negative scores in emotional content than the nonaggressive group, as well as higher, more positive scores in self-image.

One ANOVA revealed that aggressiveness was related to emotional content scores to a degree that was significant at the .01 level of probability ($F$ [1,209] = 7.06, $p$ = .01). Another ANOVA found that aggressiveness was significantly related to self-image scores ($F$ [1,209] = 3.86, $p$ = .05). A chi-square analysis indicated that aggression was related to responses that scored 1 point in emotional content together with 5 points in self-image to a highly significant degree ($\chi^2$ [1] = 27.57, $p$ <. 001). In other words, the aggressive group drew more positive perceptions of themselves and more negative perceptions of others than did the nonaggressive group.

Significant gender differences also emerged. Female students had higher scores on the emotional content scale than did male students, to a highly significant degree ($F$ [1,209) = 19.68, $p$ < .001). Male students were more likely than female students to be classified as aggressive. ($\chi^2$ [1] = 9.66, $p$ = .002) and aggressive male students had higher self-image scores than aggressive female students ($F$ [1,207] = 5.39, $p$ = .02). No significant age differences emerged.

# Questions and Implications

What is the relationship between aggressive fantasies and aggressive behavior? Were the six students in the control group who scored 1 point in emotional content together with 5 points in self-image aggressive only in fantasy? Was their aggressiveness masked, overlooked, or under control? Can we distinguish between fantasies and acting out? Do drawings about heroes reflect a desire to protect, or a masked desire to harm?

Do responses to the drawing task tend to remain stable over time, or do they reflect temporary moods? Consistencies may reflect unresolved problems and ongoing concerns, while changes may indicate that the therapeutic programs were effective. And finally, were some of the children and adolescents depressed as well as aggressive? A few students in both the aggressive and control groups scored 1 point in both emotional content and self-image.

And what is the role of humor in aggressive behavior? According to Vaillard (2002), humor may turn into passive-aggressive behavior or acting out, suggesting that the different kinds of humor expressed may provide information that is relevant. The findings, and the questions they raised, led to further investigation.

The third study examined more closely the emotional content and self-images of responses by the aggressive and nonaggressive groups (Silver, 2005). In emotional content, the aggressive group was much more negative than the nonaggressive control group. More than twice as many students in the aggressive group scored 1 point (63%) compared with the control group (30%), a difference significant at the .01 level of probability.

On the other hand, none of the aggressive students drew strongly positive fantasies, compared with 4% of the controls, and almost twice as many controls drew moderately positive fantasies scoring 4 points (12% of the controls, 7% of the aggressive group).

In self-image, however, it was the other way around. Almost three times as many aggressive students drew strongly positive self-images, with 43% scoring 5 points, compared with 15% for the controls, another difference that was significant at the .05 level of probability.

More than three times as many nonaggressive students (63%) drew fantasies that were ambivalent, ambiguous, or unclear, scoring 3 points (compared with 20% of the aggressive group).

More than four times as many aggressive students (17%) drew strongly negative self-images, scoring 1 point, compared with 4% of the controls, suggesting they may have been depressed as well as aggressive. Also in the nonaggressive control group, eight students drew strongly negative fantasies, scoring 1 point in both emotional content and self-image. None had been identified as depressed, and all were presumably typical students who had expressed interest in joining a research study.

Although students in both aggressive and control groups represented themselves as assailants, scoring 1 point in emotional content combined with 5 points in self-image, two distinctive subgroups emerged—those of predatory aggression and reactive aggression.

## Predatory Aggression, Humorous Responses, and Reactive Aggression

### Predatory Aggression

In the aggressive group, 5 of the 30 students drew assailants making unprovoked attacks on vulnerable victims, and seemed to identify with the assailants in their drawings. They were asked to respond to the drawing task on several occasions to find out if they showed consistency in the subjects they chose or the attitudes they expressed.

For example, Shaun, age 12, responded to the drawing task three times at weekly intervals. Each time he chose the stimulus drawing of a knife and drew it poised above a victim. For two of his drawings he chose the chick, which seemed to represent the victim, and the mouse, which seemed to represent himself. In his first response, "I don't like chickens! The chicken is going to die," Shaun's mouse wields a knife and smiles as he confronts the chick, as another knife descends on the chick from above (see fig. 4.1a). For his second response, he again chose the knife and added the castle. In his drawing, someone invisible throws a series of knives at a parachutist who is about to land on the castle's roof. Shaun's story was, "The castle is under attack. The guy dies" (see fig. 4.1b). For his third response, he chose the chick, knife, and mouse. The mouse smiles as the knife descends on the chick. Shaun's story was, "The bird will die" (see fig. 4.1c). Four of the five aggressive students were classmates in a school that did not provide special programs, and follow-up was not possible.

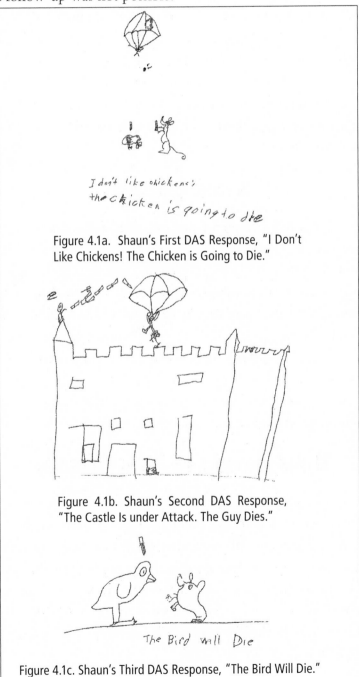

Figure 4.1a. Shaun's First DAS Response, "I Don't Like Chickens! The Chicken is Going to Die."

Figure 4.1b. Shaun's Second DAS Response, "The Castle Is under Attack. The Guy Dies."

Figure 4.1c. Shaun's Third DAS Response, "The Bird Will Die."

## Humorous Responses

In the aggressive group, the students who drew humorous responses used negative humor only, mostly lethal and morbid humor, scoring 1 point. The mean score was 1.6 points on the humor scale. In the control group, however, humor tended to be positive, the mean score being 3.3 points.

In addition, more aggressive than nonaggressive students drew humorous responses, 20% compared with 1.6% of the controls. No aggressive student used positive or ambivalent humor, and four used humor that was both lethal and morbid.

In the control group, three students drew humorous responses. One used playful humor, scoring 5 points (a man looking for a cat that is standing on his head). Two used resilient humor, scoring 4 points. For example, one drew a mouse trying to talk his way out of becoming lunch for a snake: "Don't you wanna eat the chicken?"

These findings suggest that there is an association between predatory aggression and humor that is both lethal and morbid.

## Reactive Aggression

Connor (2002) has defined reactive or defensive aggression as an angry reaction to real or perceived danger, motivated not by reward but by a need to defend against threat. Its intent is to inflict injury or pain rather than benefit the aggressor.

In the aggressive group, the responses of 5 of the 30 aggressive students suggested reactive aggression (17%) compared with none of the 181 students in the control group. For example, Toby, age 12, chose the parachutist and the knife and identified himself as a "Guy saving his girl friend. Evil guys are trying to kill him" (see fig. 4.2). Toby was overweight, teased by his peers, and had been receiving clinical assistance elsewhere because it was not provided in his school. Other schools in this study provided this assistance, as will be discussed in chapter 11.

## Masked Depression and Gender Differences

Although many of the aggressive students drew strongly positive self-images, 5 of the 30 drew strongly negative self-images, scoring 1 point on both the self-image and emotional content scales, representing themselves as victims in life-threatening situations, and suggesting that they may have been depressed. For example, Jimmy, age 14, chose four stimulus drawings: parachutist, dinosaur, volcano, and castle. His story was, "The man ejected in the war with the dinosaurs. . . . The plane was shot down by the dinosaur's breath attack. He says he is going to die because the dinosaur is in the castle" (see fig. 4.3).

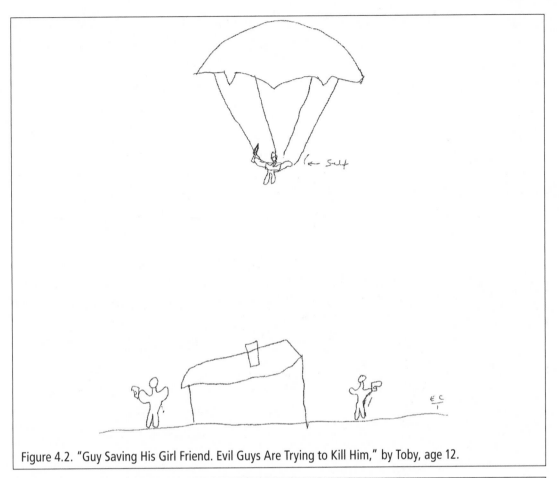

Figure 4.2. "Guy Saving His Girl Friend. Evil Guys Are Trying to Kill Him," by Toby, age 12.

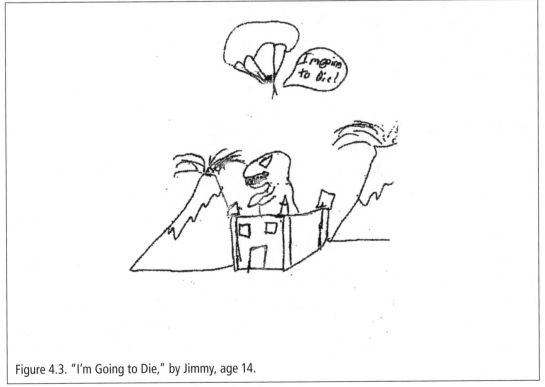

Figure 4.3. "I'm Going to Die," by Jimmy, age 14.

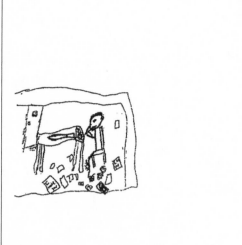

Figure 4.4. "Stress Messes with Every One . . . Just End It Forever," by a boy, age 17.

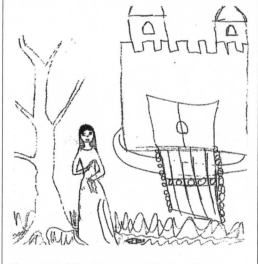

Figure 4.5. "The Prencess Kill'd Herself Because She Is Not Happy," by a girl, age 13.

In the nonaggressive control group, eight students also drew strongly negative fantasies, scoring 1 point in both emotional content and self-image; two of the eight drew solitary subjects contemplating suicide (see figs. 4.4 and 4.5). Four chose stimulus drawings with symbolic meanings: two drew chicks (one about to be sliced in half by the knife, the other having no friends and scared of people), one the barren tree (stabbed by the knife), and one the snake (trying to escape from an erupting volcano). Five chose and drew the stimulus drawing knife, and two the volcano, and all were fantasies about solitary living subjects.

None had been identified as depressed, and all were presumably typical students attending regular classes in their schools who happened to respond to the drawing task because their parents had granted permission for them to participate in a research study. (Since their parents had granted permission for them to participate anonymously, it was not possible to alert their parents or refer them for clinical follow-up in their schools.)

The 13 students in both groups who scored 1 point on both scales also drew fantasies about life-threatening situations. Eleven drew hostile environments, 7 were helpless, and 3 were calling for help. Eight seemed hopeless and doomed to die. Six chose and drew the stimulus drawing knife; five, the volcano; and four, the castle.

Other differences between the aggressive and nonaggressive students emerged. None in the aggressive group drew suicidal fantasies, and none seemed to represent themselves as sad or fearful, whereas four in the control group drew solitary subjects that were crying, holding handkerchiefs, or exposed to rain. No boys in the aggressive group chose the chick as their only live subject, perhaps because the term *chicken* is synonymous with *cowardice*. Perhaps those in the aggressive group had become assailants in order to deny or conceal fear, anger, or despair.

The emotional content and self-images that emerged in the responses of these 13 aggressive and nonaggressive children and adolescents match those of patients hospitalized with clinical depression in previous studies, and suggest that they were suffering from masked depression.

## Male Responses

Throughout human history and across cultures, males have been hunters and warriors, and it might be expected that males tend to fantasize about assaultive relationships, as found in the present study as well as in previous studies of gender differences in responses to the drawing task (Silver, 1992, 1993a, 1996c). As Connor (2002) has observed, aggression tends to be reinforced in boys because it is generally seen as masculine, whereas girls experience pressures from parents, teachers, and peers to conform to stereotypes of feminine behavior that tend to suppress aggression.

Other investigators have observed that male aggressiveness tends to be physical, overt, and direct, whereas female aggression tends to be indirect, covert, and relational, making it harder to observe and quantify (Bjorkqvist, Osterman, & Kaukianen, 1992). Indirect aggression protects the aggressor from retaliation and induces others to attack victims. In addition, female aggressiveness has been correlated with sexual abuse, delinquency, conduct disorder, family dysfunction, depression, and anxiety. The pilot study of aggressive and nonaggressive children and adolescents found that gender was significantly related to aggressiveness.

In the present study, only boys and adolescents expressed predatory aggression, all were covert, and all were in the aggressive group. According to Carl, the dinosaur did it; Ramon blamed the volcano; and in the drawings by Shaun, Sam, and Gus, the stabbers and knife throwers were invisible.

## Female Responses

In the aggressive group, 5 of the 30 students were girls, but 3 of the 5 seemed to represent themselves as victims rather than assailants, using symbols and metaphors to represent themselves and/or their assailants indirectly. One chose the princess/bride and the snake, drawing the princess with no arms and the snake attacking her groin. Another chose the parachutist and the knife, changed the parachute into an empty balloon, crossed out "girl" and wrote, "The balloon was cut with a knife and into the sea and was never found." Both responses are consistent with the observations that female aggressiveness tends to be indirect and correlated with sexual abuse. A third girl seemed to identify with the stimulus drawing chick she transformed into a large, scowling hen defending a small mouse, expressing reactive aggression. A fourth seemed to have four self-images, both overt (the passive princess "stuck in a castle") and covert (volcano about to explode, cat chasing mouse, and chick killing snake).

Although responses to the drawing task support the observation that aggression is more prevalent among males, they fail to support the observation that indirect and covert aggression is more prevalent among females. Both genders tended to be indirect and covert, disguising their victims as well as their assailants.

In the control group, the female mean score was higher, more positive, than the male mean score in both emotional content (2.83 female, 2.24 male) and self-image (3.44 female, 2.94 male). In emotional content, more than twice as many girls drew fantasies with positive emotional content (42%, compared with 20% of the boys).

A total of 5 of the 85 girls, but none of the 96 boys, scored 5 points in both emotional content and self-image, and all chose the stimulus drawings of the princess and the castle. Of the 5 girls, 4 mentioned princes or grooms in their stories but failed to include them in their drawings.

Also in the control group, 20 of the 85 girls chose and drew both princess and castle (24%), and 15 of the 20 expressed negative emotional content. To illustrate, one princess, who lived in a palace, "was so beautiful that no one was allowed to see her so she was always by herself and never got married. She lived sadly ever after by herself." Another princess was "running away because of the people who told her what to do. She made a rope down her room when she ran into the forest when a snake gets her. Who will save her now." As discussed previously, another princess was stabbed to death, and two committed suicide.

On the other hand, two of the girls in the control group who chose the princess and the castle drew strongly positive fantasies, scoring 5 points in both emotional content and self-image. Although one princess seemed quite stout, she was described as beautiful, very happy, and romantically involved with a handsome prince.

Seven girls, but no boys, drew strongly positive fantasies about happy solitary subjects or loving relationships, scoring 5 points in emotional content, whereas 18% of the boys, compared with 11% of the girls, seemed to identify with powerful and effective subjects, scoring 5 points in self-image.

Substantial gender differences also emerged among those scoring 3.5 and 4 points: 14 boys, but only 1 girl, drew ambivalent fantasies with positive outcomes, scoring 3.5 points; and 18% of the girls, compared with only 1% of the boys, seemed to identify with fortunate but passive subjects or friendly relationships, scoring 4 points.

Comparing girls in the aggressive and nonaggressive control groups, the self-image scores of the aggressive girls were lower (more negative than positive), their mean score being 2.6, whereas the mean score of the nonaggressive girls (3.2) was higher (more positive than negative). Comparing the groups of boys, self-images in the aggressive group were more positive, their mean scores 3.8, whereas the mean score of the non-aggressive boys was more negative, at 3.2. Larger gender differences emerged in the self-image mean scores in the aggressive group but not the nonaggressive group, where both genders scored 3.2 points. In emotional content, the gender differences were reversed; the boys were much more negative.

How can these findings be explained? Why did the aggressive girls have more negative self-images than the nonaggressive girls, and the aggressive boys more positive self-images than the nonaggressive boys? Are the differences biological? Are they cultural? A study of responses to the DAS assessment from delinquent and nondelinquent girls and boys in Russia is presented in chapter 12.

Do two or more responses to the drawing task clarify intentions, meanings, and emotional states? Presenting the drawing task again on another day could clarify the question whether a strongly negative fantasy reflects a passing mood or persistent emotional state. In addition, changes in positive or negative scores could reflect changes in circumstances or the effectiveness of programs. On the other hand, consistencies in the choice of stimulus drawings, symbols, self-image, and relationships between the subjects portrayed could illuminate anxieties and coping strategies. Consistencies across multiple responses after intervals of time could also support the reliability of the DAS assessment.

## Additional Findings and Observations

None of the aggressive students expressed moderately negative views of self and the world, scoring 2 points on both scales. One student scored 2 points in self-image, but then scored 1 point in emotional content, portraying himself as running away from life-threatening danger. Another scored 2 points in emotional content (hostile relationships) but 5 in self-image.

Nine students (30%) scored 3 points in emotional content, self-image, or both. Fifteen (50%) drew wish-fulfilling fantasies, and 3 of the 15 were moderately positive, scoring 4 points. Twelve of the 15 (40%) represented themselves as powerful and effective, with 6 drawing homicidal fantasies—lethal encounters in which the murderers seemed to be themselves. One student represented himself as an exploding volcano; another, as an aggressive mouse. Four portrayed themselves as heroes protecting victims.

## The Silver Drawing Test and Draw a Story

The findings seem to indicate that the DAS assessment shows promise as a means to identify students at risk for aggressive behavior. The aggressive group, when compared with the nonaggressive group, drew more fantasies about homicidal and life-threatening situations, and drew themselves as powerful and effective. They had significantly lower scores in emotional content (1 point) and higher scores in self-image (5 points). These findings raised questions with implications for clinicians and educators, and suggest that further investigation would be worthwhile.

# Chapter 5

# Using Draw a Story with Clinical and Nonclinical Populations

◇   ◇   ◇

This chapter reviews additional studies that used the Draw a Story (DAS) assessment for different purposes. It also suggests procedures to facilitate the identification of students who may be at risk for aggression and/or depression. The studies compare the responses of adolescents with and without emotional disturbances, age and gender differences in attitudes toward self and others, and gender differences in the fantasies of adolescents with and without histories of delinquent behavior. They also include studies by various practitioners who used DAS with clinical and nonclinical populations.

## Adolescents with and without Emotional Disturbances

This study compared responses to DAS Form A by 95 adolescents who had been diagnosed previously as having emotional disturbances with 68 presumably nondisturbed adolescents who served as controls. The adolescents, ages 13 to 17, included four subgroups: 35 girls with disturbances, 60 boys with disturbances, 42 control girls, and 26 control boys. Thirteen art therapists or teachers administered the DAS assessment to the disturbed students in special schools, special classes in public schools, or psychiatric facilities in Florida, Georgia, Nebraska, New York, and Oregon. Six art therapists or teachers administered it to the control students in four public schools and one private school in Florida, Minnesota, New York, and Ohio. Madeline Altabe, PhD, used chi-square analyses to determine the proportions of each group in obtaining certain scores.

## Results

Significant differences were found between the groups. As might be expected, fewer disturbed adolescents responded with positive themes, scored 4 and 5 points ($\chi^2$ [1] = 13.26). Girls in the normal control group had the most positive scores (43%) followed by disturbed boys (26%), boys in the normal control group (16%), and disturbed girls (14%).

Twice as many adolescents in the control group drew strongly positive fantasies about caring relationships or effective solitary subjects, scoring 5 points (18% controls, 9% disturbed). More than six times as many control girls as control boys scored 5 points (26%, vs 4%), and about twice as many disturbed boys than girls scored 5 points (20%, vs 11%), as shown in table 5.1.

Table 5.1    Comparing DAS Scores of 95 Adolescents with Disturbances, Ages 13 to 16, with 68 Controls

| Adolescents | Mean | 1 pt | 2 pts | 3 pts | 4 pts | 5 pts |
|---|---|---|---|---|---|---|
| 68 control | 2.39 | 40% | 18% | 10% | 15% | 18% |
| 95 disturbed | 2.25 | 36% | 31% | 21% | 3% | 9% |
| 42 control girls, | 2.88 | 31% | 19% | 7% | 17% | 26% |
| 26 control boys | 1.89 | 54% | 15% | 15% | 12% | 4% |
| 35 girls with disturbance | 2.43 | 26% | 31% | 29% | 3% | 11% |
| 60 boys with disturbance | 2.07 | 20% | 29% | 24% | 6% | 20% |

The normal control groups drew fantasies about friendly relationships (4 points), or fortunate but passive solitary subjects, five times more often than adolescents with disturbances (15% of control, 3% of disturbed). Even greater differences emerged between the two groups of girls (17% of controls, 3% of girls with disturbances). This difference also was statistically significant ($\chi^2$ [1] = 9.8). Although more control boys than boys with disturbances scored 4 points, only twice as many did so (12%, vs 6%), which is not significant.

In negative responses, boys in the control group had most of the strongly negative scores (1 point). This result was also significant ($\chi^2$ [1] = 4.88). No significant differences were found between the girls who drew moderately negative responses scoring 2 points.

There were no significant patterns within the groups for a score of 2, 3, or 4 points. The pattern of results for 5 points (control girls more positive than emotionally disturbed girls) was significant ($\chi^2$ [1] = 16.72).

## Observations

It was surprising to find the disturbed girls less inclined to portray friendly relationships or fortunate solitary subjects than girls in the control group, to significant degrees. It was also surprising that no significant differences emerged between the two groups in portraying stressful relationships or unfortunate solitary subjects. The finding suggests that the absence of positive themes may be more meaningful than the presence of negative themes. The finding that the presumably normal boys drew fantasies about assaultive relationships significantly more often than the disturbed boys did is less surprising because similar findings emerged in previous studies (Silver, 1993a and 1996b). The paucity of positive scores may prove more useful than the prevalence of negative scores in screening for emotional disturbances or masked depression.

# Age and Gender Differences in Attitudes toward Self and Others

This study was undertaken, in part, because it had been reported that males tend to focus on independence and competition, whereas females focus on relationships and caring for others (Gilligan, Ward, Taylor, & Bardige, 1988; Tannen, 1990). These investigators had relied on verbal communication. Would responses to the DAS assessment provide similar information?

DAS responses by 360 children, adolescents, and adults were separated into drawings about solitary subjects and drawings about relationships, assigned to age and gender groups, and scored on the rating scale (Silver, 1993b). Age and gender groups were then compared.

The respondents included 203 females and 157 males in five age groups: children ages 9 to 12; younger adolescents, ages 13 to 16; older adolescents, ages 17 to 19; younger adults, ages 21 to 64; and adults, age 65 or older. The 56 children included 32 girls and 24 boys. Thirty-three had been diagnosed as emotionally disturbed (ED) or learning disabled (LD), 14 were hospitalized as clinically depressed, and 9 were presumably normal. The 147 younger adolescents included 71 girls and 76 boys. Thirteen were hospitalized patients with depression, 78 had been diagnosed as ED or LD and attended special schools, and 56 were unimpaired. The 68 older adolescents included 30 girls and 38 boys: 1 hospitalized for clinical depression, 27 diagnosed as ED or LD, and 40 unimpaired. The 79 adults included 7 hospitalized women with depression, 53 nondepressed women, and 19 men. Thirteen art therapists in 10 states—Arizona, Florida, Georgia, Maine, Montana, New Jersey, New York, Ohio, Pennsylvania, and Washington—volunteered to administer the DAS assessment.

## Results

In drawings about solitary subjects, no gender differences emerged. Both males and females expressed more negative than positive attitudes toward the subjects they portrayed. Across the five female age groups, 41% of the responses portrayed sad or helpless (1 point) or angry or fearful subjects (2 points), compared with 28% who drew fantasies about passive or active pleasures (4 and 5 points). Across male age groups, 49% scored 1 and 2 points, compared with 27% who scored 4 and 5 points. The young boys expressed the most negative attitudes, 75% scoring 1 point, whereas none of the girls scored 1 point. The older women were the most positive: 41% drawing solitary subjects engaged in active pleasures, and 12% in passive pleasures.

In drawings about relationships, however, gender differences emerged. Male responses tended to be more negative—72% portraying assaultive and stressful relationships, compared with 34% of the females. On the other hand, 9% of the males and 29% of the females portrayed friendly and caring relationships. The most negative relationships appeared in drawings by boys (80%), younger adolescents (75%), and older adolescents (67%), whereas female relationships tended to be mixed (34% negative, 29% positive, 37% neutral).

More positive relationships appeared in drawings by older women than any other age or gender group, with 46% scoring 4 or 5 points. Proportionally more women than men portrayed active solitary pleasures (41% women, 20% men). Proportionally more adolescent girls than any other female age group drew fantasies about sad, helpless, or isolated solitary subjects, scoring 1 point (35% of girls ages 13 to 16, 43% of those ages 17 to 19), as well as stressful relationships, scoring 2 points (30% of those ages 13 to 16, 38% of those ages 17 to 19).

These findings are inconsistent with the observation that females tend to focus on relationships and responsibility to others and males on independence and detachment. More males than females portrayed relationships, and both genders drew relationships more often than they drew solitary subjects.

## Sex Differences in the Solitary and Assaultive Fantasies of Delinquent and Nondelinquent Adolescents

Self-images expressed in response to the DAS assessment were examined for differences in gender, age, and delinquency (Silver, 1996b). The subjects included 64 adolescents in detention in California and 74 normal controls attending schools in New York, Ohio, and Florida; 82 were male (53 delinquent, 29 controls) and 56 were female (11 delinquent, 45 controls). Their ages ranged from 13 to 17. The responses were divided into four groups: gender, delinquency, drawings about solitary subjects, and drawings about relationships. Mean scores were analyzed and compared.

The first analysis asked whether gender or delinquency was related to self-image scores—that is, to fortunate, unfortunate, or aggressive self-image. No significant differences emerged. The male mean score was 2.52; the female mean score, 2.92.

The second analysis asked whether the proportions of drawings about solitary subjects or assaultive relationships differed, depending on delinquency or gender. Significant gender differences emerged in both solitary and assaultive content, and the finding of assaultive content was reversed for solitary content. Overall, males and females differed in both aggressive content ($\chi^2$ [1] = 11.00, $p < .01$) and solitary content ($\chi^2$ [1] = 6.33; $p < .05$); 31.7% of the males drew pictures about assaultive relationships, compared with 5.4% of the females.

In solitary content, however, 37.5% of the females drew pictures about solitary subjects, compared with 15.9% of the males. Solitary content also distinguished between delinquent and control groups: 33.8% of the control subjects drew solitary subjects as compared with 14.1% of the subjects who were delinquent.

The differences in assaultive content found in drawings by delinquent and control male and female adolescents reached significance ($\chi^2$ [1] = 9.11; $p < .01$). The difference between delinquent males and females, however, did not reach significance (28.3% of the males drew assaultive relationships; no females who were delinquent drew assaultive relationships). Although males in the control group differed significantly from females in the control group, males who were delinquent did not differ significantly from females who were delinquent.

Control group males used aggressive humor in 45.4% of their assaultive drawings, but aggressive humor did not emerge in any other group. A group (delinquent vs control) by gender (male vs female) two-by-two analysis of variance was conducted on the self-image rating. No significant results were found.

In drawings about solitary subjects, gender differences were large in the control group, small in the delinquent group. When negative attitudes toward solitary subjects were examined, gender differences emerged in both delinquent and control groups. Proportionally more females than males drew sad or helpless solitary subjects (delinquent females, 18.1%; control females, 17.8%; delinquent males, 9.4%; control males, 6.9%).

When positive attitudes toward solitary subjects were examined, control groups predominated (control females, 20%; control males, 13.8%; delinquent males, 3.7%; delinquent females, 0).

The gender difference was large in the control group but small in the delinquent group. Drawings by delinquent females were more like the male drawings of both groups. Thus, greater gender differences were found in the normal control groups than among delinquent adolescents.

To summarize, no differences in gender or delinquency were found when mean scores were examined, but differences appeared when drawings about assaultive relationships or solitary subjects were examined. Gender made a difference in negative responses scored 1 and 2 points. More than twice as many females as males drew sad or helpless solitary subjects (18% of females and 8% of males). Delinquency also made a difference in positive responses scored 4 and 5 points. Nondelinquent males outnumbered delinquent males (14% vs 4%) in portraying fortunate subjects. No delinquent females, but 20% of the controls, drew fortunate subjects. The effect was reversed for aggressive content. Delinquent females were more like males, regardless of delinquency.

As found in the previous study, more nondelinquent than delinquent males drew fantasies about assaultive relationships. Perhaps the difference can be explained by the difference between fantasizing about violence and acting violently, or it may be that incarceration inhibits the expression of aggressive fantasies.

The finding that no females who were delinquent expressed positive feelings toward their solitary self-images suggests that they may be more at risk, or that incarceration dimmed or extinguished their wish-fulfilling fantasies. On the other hand, the sample may have been too small.

---

### Identifying Students at Risk for Aggression and/or Depression

1. Identify respondents who score 1 point in both emotional content and self-image, as well as those who score 1 point in emotional content combined with 5 points in self-image when responding to either the DAS assessment or the Silver Drawing Test (SDT) Drawing from Imagination task.

2. Discuss the responses individually and privately with the individuals who drew them, whenever possible, to clarify intended and unintended meanings.

3. Score each response for emotional content, self-image, and, when appropriate, the use of humor and level of cognitive skills.

4. Collect information about the respondent's family history and relationships with peers and teachers, as well as normal and atypical development and behavior.

5. Ask the respondents to respond to the DAS or SDT Form B set of stimulus drawings on two or more occasions, reserving Form A for posttesting at the end of the program.

6. Establish programs as needed: preventive programs for reactive aggression and for predatory aggression, as well as therapeutic programs for depression and/or reactive aggression.

7. Keep responses on file to review and compare with subsequent responses in order to note changes and consistencies.

---

## Ellison's Use of DAS with Delinquent Adolescents

Joanne Ellison, ATR-BC, investigated the possible benefits of using DAS to provide rapid assessment of young male offenders in a probation camp, so that more accurate and timely mental health referrals could be made (Silver & Ellison, 1995, part 2). She found very little resistance, in part because of the structured setting, but for some, she noted, "it was like giving food to the starving." She observed that DAS circumvented stereotyping and written components with symbolic pictures that provide clues to intentions. She illustrated these and other observations with case studies. She also observed that many of her clients were more kinesthetic than verbal, that sad and aggressive stories may indicate depression, and that happy fantasies may indicate denial on the part of youths who are equally depressed and who may be more resistant to treatment.

Ellison concluded that a structured art assessment such as DAS can be useful in the evaluation of juveniles with conduct disorders. Their drawings can help us understand the concerns and occasionally the underlying dynamics of these individuals.

## Turner's Use of DAS with Adolescents Who Experienced Abuse

Christine Turner, ATR-BC (1993), used DAS with adolescent clients in a psychiatric hospital as one of a series of five assessments to assess possible history of abuse. She found it useful in assessing the extent of abuse, the meaning attached to abuse, and the effects of abuse on her clients' defenses, coping skills, sense of self, relationships, and worldview. She then made treatment recommendations to assist ward therapists in working with clients, and for aftercare, as needed.

Turner asked her clients to respond to five requests: free subject, scribble drawing, kinetic family drawing, self-drawing, and DAS Form A, placing DAS last because she found that its more cognitive nature provided closure.

The emerging themes often confirmed impressions derived from the preceding four drawings and other sources. Occasionally, however, the adolescent who had produced four guarded, stereotypical images experienced greater freedom in working with the DAS cartoon figures and metaphorical storytelling. Conversely, the client who accessed and expressed painful feelings might use DAS to "regroup" and condense the content of the other four drawings into a safely distanced metaphor.

The client's areas of greatest need are often graphically depicted in responses to DAS. Cognitive schemas relating to the need may also be apparent. Beliefs concerning attribution of causality, locus of control, concerns about self-protective abilities, trust and mistrust, self-value, and community attachments suggested by DAS responses became topics for discussion in the assessment interviews. In discussing with clients that they can stay with the metaphor while exploring trauma-related themes, therapists have the opportunity to begin addressing treatment needs, confirming reality, and laying the groundwork for future therapy.

## Wilson's Use of DAS with Patients Who Had Brain Injuries

Mary Wilson, ATR (1993), used DAS Form A to assess the emotional outlook and skills of inpatients and outpatients who had sustained brain injuries in accidents, assaults, strokes, or aneurysms. To assess word-finding difficulty, identification skills, and speaking ability, she presented the stimulus drawings mounted on a cardboard background, asking patients to identify each image. To assess ability to establish relationships and to create and organize images, she noted the patient's ability to combine subjects and show something happening between them. She also examined executive functioning, reasoning, problem-solving abilities, and field-neglect problems, which became evident if the patient drew closer to one side of the page or the other. During the story-writing stage of the task, she observed reading and writing skills.

As a member of the clinical treatment team trying to assess a patient's strengths and weaknesses, Wilson found that DAS served to reinforce the findings of other therapists and in many instances contributed information about emotional outlook, depression, and fantasies. She found that patients almost always projected themselves into their drawings and stories, offering material about their emotional inner lives. They revealed issues of low self-esteem, concerns about adjustment to disability, and depression over losses.

Wilson (1990) also used the assessment with hospitalized adolescents who were depressed and suicidal. She administered it during the first session of a biweekly treatment program and again months later to gain insight into changes in emotional outlook and how the sense of self and environment were evolving. Of 13 respondents, 12 drew pictures about negative or severely frightening events. Only one response was positive. Wilson found the task useful for assessing her patients' emotional states and how they viewed their situations.

## Dunn-Snow's Use of DAS with Emotionally Disturbed Children and Adolescents

Peggy Dunn-Snow, ATR-BC (1994), used DAS Form A to assess the needs of students who were diagnosed with severe emotional disturbances but were able to attend elementary and secondary schools in a large urban school district. She also adapted DAS for use as a therapeutic technique, presenting a case study in which she used the task to determine whether a high school student was depressed. After the student responded with self-destructive thoughts, she checked school records and discovered he had a history of clinical depression; she then used the task to help him resolve feelings about the death of his father.

Dunn-Snow also used DAS in working with students who became anxious when asked to do relatively free-choice artwork. She found that it provided a second grader with sufficient structure and support to begin making art, and it broke down resistance among students who previously refused to participate.

In addition, Dunn-Snow adapted DAS for group therapy and to resolve conflicts. In working with fifth-grade boys, she used it to provide structure and set limits, inviting each boy to choose a subject, then collaborate with others in the group by combining their images into a single drawing with a common theme, title, and story line. She noted that in accomplishing this task, her students followed directions, accepted limits, solved problems, made compromises, and communicated effectively.

## Coffey's Use of DAS in a Psychiatric Hospital

C. M. Coffey, in her master's thesis (1995), found that male and female patients in the psychiatric units of two hospitals seemed to have different needs and suggested that gender be considered in planning therapeutic treatment. Males seemed more reticent to reveal themselves to anyone. Females seemed less apt to recognize their rights or self-worth and were fearful that moving toward one goal foreclosed other goals. Some patients were very agitated, some abused equipment or themselves, and others displayed a heavy, pervasive sadness. She observed that projective drawing appeared less threatening to evasive or resistant patients than tests like the Thematic Apperception Test or the Rorschach, and served to establish rapport, uncover areas of patient interests, indicate abilities, and reveal defense mechanisms.

## Brandt's Use of DAS with Adolescents—
## Sex Offenders, the Depressed, and the Typical

Michele Brandt, in her master's thesis (1995), examined the importance of visual arts in assessing and treating adolescents who committed sex offenses, comparing them with typical adolescents and adolescents who were depressed. Participating in her study were 14 males in a residential facility who committed sex offenses, ages 12 to 18, with the average age being 16 years. She compared their mean score on DAS (1.89) with the mean scores of typical adolescents (2.73) and adolescents with depression (3.14). The findings suggested that those committing sex offenses are likely to be depressed and to perceive themselves and their world in negative ways. They also suggested that art expression enables those who work with adolescents committing sex offenses to tap into emotionality and therefore is useful in treatment programs that emphasize cognition and behavior.

## Observations

The new studies of depression and aggression support and amplify the findings of previous studies, suggesting that the DAS assessment can provide a useful tool for access to fantasies and feelings about self and others as well as for identifying children and adolescents who may be depressed or potentially violent. They also suggest that this assesment could be used not only by art therapists and other mental health professionals but also by elementary and secondary school teachers who could refer students at risk to clinicians or administrators for further assessment.

# Section II

# The Silver Drawing Test: Drawing What You Predict, What You See, and What You Imagine

◇    ◇    ◇

# Chapter 6

# Why and How the Silver Drawing Test Was Developed and Field Tested

◇     ◇     ◇

Originally, the Silver Drawing Test (SDT) was designed to bypass language disabilities by assessing cognitive skills through drawings. It evolved from a belief that we tend to underestimate the intelligence of children like Charlie, who at age 11 could not hear, speak, lip-read, or read words, but could read a floor plan of the Metropolitan Museum of Art even when it was upside down in my hand, and he led the way when our art class visited the museum. He showed extraordinary skill in drawing.

Although the psychologist in his school claimed that Charlie's intelligence could not be tested, I wrote to a distinguished psychologist, E. Paul Torrance, who sent a copy of his Torrance Test of Creative Thinking, Figural Form A, and offered to score the results.

Compared with children who did not have disabilities, Charlie scored in the upper 5% in originality, the upper 3% in fluency, the upper 10% in flexibility, and in elaboration was "almost unexcelled." As Torrance wrote, his performance was "truly outstanding" and reflected "a high order of ability to acquire information, form relationships, and in general, to think."

The psychologist in Charlie's school was not impressed. She said, "it changes nothing" because "language comes first, and there's a limit to what you can do without language."

What are the limits? My search for answers led eventually to the SDT.

The SDT includes three subtests: Drawing from Imagination, Predictive Drawing, and Drawing from Observation. Each subtest was designed to assess one of the three fundamental and independent structures of knowledge from which all branches of knowledge can be generated (Piaget, 1970). The first is based on the concept of a group and applies to classes and numbers. The second is based on the idea of sequential order and applies to relationships. The third is based on ideas of space and applies to neighborhoods, points of view, and frames of reference. Although these ideas may seem highly abstract, Piaget has observed similar ideas in the thinking of children as young as 6 or 7, and although the concepts are usually associated with language, they can also be perceived and expressed visually.

The same concepts seem to be fundamental in reading. In examining the performances of children with dyslexia on the Wechsler Intelligence Scale for Children (see, e.g., Wechsler, 2003), or WISC, Bannatyne (1971) noted that they performed well on WISC subtests involving spatial ability, moderately well on subtests of conceptual ability, and poorly on subtests of sequential ability. He also observed that these children had intellectual abilities of a visual-spatial nature that are seldom recognized or trained. Other investigators also found that readers with disabilities scored highest in the spatial category and lowest in the sequential category (Rugel, 1974; Smith, Coleman, Dokecki, & Davis, 1977).

The subtests are also based on the ability to conserve, to recognize that an object remains the same in spite of transformations in its appearance. Most rational thought depends on conservation, according to Piaget (1970), and Bruner and colleagues (1966) noted that the ability to recognize equivalence under different guises is a powerful idea not only in science but in everyday life. Up to the age of about 7, children typically are unable to conserve a quantity of liquid over alterations in its appearance.

## The SDT Tasks: Drawing from Imagination, Predictive Drawing, and Drawing from Observation

### Drawing from Imagination

As discussed in chapter 1, respondents are asked to select stimulus drawings, imagine something happening between them, and then draw what they imagine. As they finish drawing, they are asked to add titles or stories and, finally, to discuss their responses whenever possible. The task is based on the observation that different individuals perceive the same stimulus drawing differently, that past experiences influence their perceptions, and that their responses reflect cognitive skills and facets of personality that can be quantified.

This SDT task provides two sets of stimulus drawings. Form A includes 15 stimulus drawings reserved for pretesting and posttesting only. Responses to Form A were used in the studies of reliability and validity presented in chapter 8 and to collect the normative data presented in chapter 9. Form B is provided for use in therapeutic and developmental programs. Both forms are reproduced in appendix A.

Responses to the drawing task usually have two components, cognitive and emotional, and both are assessed on rating scales that range from 1 to 5 points.

## Cognitive Content

Selecting, combining, and representing seem to be fundamental not only in cognition but also in the visual arts, neurobiology, and linguistics. Painters, for example, select and combine colors or shapes, and when their work is representational, they select, combine, and represent images as well.

The neurobiologist Semir Zeki (1999) has observed that the visual arts contribute to our understanding of the visual brain because they explore and reveal the brain's perceptual capabilities (Zeki, 2001). The brain searches for constancies, and distills the essential characters of objects and situations from successive views (Zeki, 1999). It is a collection of many different anatomical areas and individual cells, which are highly selective for particular attributes, such as straight lines, but indifferent to other lines. By selecting and rejecting, the brain forms categories that integrate and represent many objects and many situations. Zeki notes that the visual arts also seek constancies, and they contribute to understanding because they explore and reveal the brain's perceptual capabilities.

The linguist Ramon Jakobson (1964) has identified selecting and combining as the two fundamental verbal operations. The ability to produce language begins with selecting words, then combines the words into sentences. The ability to comprehend language proceeds in the reverse order. Jakobson defines expressive language disorders as a disturbance in the ability to combine parts into wholes, and receptive language disorders as a disturbance in the ability to select.

### The Ability to Select

J.J. Hornsby, a psychologist, found three levels of ability to select (see Bruner et al., 1966). The lowest level is perceptual; the intermediate level, functional; and the highest level, abstract. In her experiments, Hornsby asked children to select objects that were alike in some way and then to explain why they were alike. The children progressed from grouping objects based on perceptual attributes, such as color or shape, to grouping based on function—what they do or what is done to them. She found that grouping based on perceptual attributes declined steadily from 47% at age 6 to 20% at age 11, whereas functional grouping increased from 30% at age 6 to 47% at age 11. She also observed that adolescents develop true conceptual grouping based on abstract, invisible attributes, such as the concept of class inclusion.

The Drawing from Imagination task is based on the premise that respondents whose drawings imply more than is visible, or who use abstract words in their titles or stories, have developed the ability to select at the abstract level (5 points), and that lower levels, based on perceptual attributes or functional grouping, can also be inferred and scored. Responses that simply show what subjects do or what can be done to them score 3 points, reflecting ability to select at the functional level, and responses with a single subject or several subjects unrelated in size or placement score 1 point, reflecting ability to select at the perceptual level. Responses at intermediate levels score 2 or 4 points.

## The Ability to Combine

The importance of being able to integrate or combine the subjects of a drawing meaningfully becomes evident when the ability is lost as a consequence of lesions in particular areas of the brain (Zeki, 1999, p. 74). Some patients can recognize the details of a face, such as the eyes or a nose, but cannot combine the information sufficiently to recognize the face of a friend or close relative. The failure is one of binding the elements together, then registering them with the brain's stored memory for that face.

Piaget and Inhelder (1967) have observed that the most rudimentary spatial relationships are based on proximity. Before the age of 7, children typically regard objects in isolation rather than as part of a comprehensive system. Gradually, they consider objects in relation to neighboring objects and to external frames of reference, such as the ground. Children tend to represent the ground by drawing or implying a baseline parallel to the bottom of the paper, relating objects to one another along this line, but as they mature they become aware of distances and proportions.

In the Drawing from Imagination task, scoring is based on the premise that responses that depict depth or take into account the whole drawing area reflect high levels of ability to combine (5 points). Responses that relate subjects to one another along a baseline reflect moderate levels of ability (3 points), and those that relate subjects on the basis of proximity reflect low levels of ability (1 point).

## The Ability to Represent (Creativity)

Drawing and painting, whether narrative or abstract, have tended to represent objects, throughout history and around the world. Children can recognize a circle long before they can draw one, as Piaget and Inhelder (1967) have pointed out. To draw a circle, a child must be able to visualize it when it is out of sight.

The ability to represent is imitative and passive at first, then intellectually active. Highly creative representations show originality, independence, and the ability to toy with ideas (Torrance, 1980). In addition, Torrance cautioned against trying to separate creativity from intelligence because they interact and overlap. He also observed that highly creative children often have inferior verbal skills.

In the SDT, scoring for the ability to represent is based on the premise that respondents whose drawings *transform* the stimulus drawings they select by being highly original, expressive, playful, or suggestive score 5 points. Responses that reveal ability to *restructure* by changing or elaborating on stimulus drawings or stereotypes score 3 points, and responses that are *imitative*—that is, simply copy stimulus drawings or use stereotypes such as stick figures—score 1 point.

## Emotional Content

Responses to the Drawing from Imagination task often reflect wishes, fears, frustrations, and conflicts, as well as inner resources such as resilience and self-disparaging humor. Strongly negative themes, such as fantasies about murderous relationships or sad solitary subjects, score 1 point. Moderately negative themes, such as fantasies about stressful relationships or frightened solitary subjects, score 2 points. The 3-point intermediate score is used for themes that are ambivalent (both negative and positive), ambiguous (unclear), or unemotional. Those that suggest negative outcomes score 2.5 points, whereas those that suggest positive outcomes score 3.5 points. The 4-point score is used to characterize moderately positive themes, such as friendly relationships or fortunate solitary subjects, and 5 points is used for strongly positive themes, such as loving relationships or powerful solitary subjects. Guidelines for scoring are presented in chapter 2, together with examples of scored responses.

Because the emotional projection scale does not distinguish between self-images and fantasies about others (which may conflict), a 5-point self-image scale is also provided. Respondents who seem to identify with subjects they portray as sad, isolated, or in mortal danger score 1 point; when their protagonists are frustrated, frightened, or unfortunate they score 2 points. Fortunate protagonists score 4 points; powerful, effective, or beloved protagonists score 5 points. Self-images that are ambivalent, ambiguous, unemotional, or invisible (such as the narrator) score 3 points.

# Predictive Drawing

In this subtest, respondents are asked to predict changes in the appearance of objects by adding lines to outline drawings. The ability to recognize that an object remains the same in spite of changes in its appearance—the ability to conserve—is basic in logical thinking (Bruner et al., 1966; Piaget, 1967). Until the age of about 7, children are unable to conserve or place objects in order systematically. Responses are scored on 5-point scales, ranging from low to high levels of ability to predict and represent concepts of sequential order as well as concepts of horizontality and verticality.

## The Concept of Sequential Order

The aim of the first task is to determine whether a respondent has acquired the ability to predict and represent a sequence. The task presents a series of line drawings of an ice cream soda and six empty glasses and asks the respondent to draw lines in the empty glasses to show how the soda would appear if gradually consumed through a straw. It is based on the premise that a respondent who draws a descending series of horizontal lines in the glasses, without corrections, has acquired the ability to order a sequence systematically (scored 5 points). Erasures and other corrections suggest that the concept has been achieved through trial and error rather than systematically, reflecting a lower level of ability. A drawing that does not represent a sequence of lines suggests that the respondent has not acquired the concept of sequential order.

The other two tasks of the Predictive Drawing subtest are designed to assess concepts of horizontality and verticality and are based on observations by Piaget and Inhelder (1967, pp. 375–385).

## The Concept of Horizontality

Zeki (1999) has proposed that lines of particular orientation are genetically determined. Piaget and Inhelder (1967) have proposed that the most stable framework of everyday experience involves horizontals and verticals. They point out that we are so used to thinking in terms of horizontals and verticals that they may seem self-evident; but when asked to draw water in bottles, children at age 4 or 5 tend to scribble round shapes. As they grow older, they draw lines parallel to the base even when the bottle is tilted; then begin to draw oblique lines, which become less oblique and more horizontal until, around the age of 9, they tend to draw horizontal lines immediately.

To determine whether respondents have acquired the ability to represent horizontality in spite of changes in appearance, the task presents outline drawings of an upright and a tilted bottle and asks respondents to draw lines in the bottles to show how the bottles would appear if half filled with water. The task is based on the premise that an individual who draws a horizontal line in the tilted bottle has learned that the surface of water remains horizontal regardless of the tilt of its container, scoring 5 points. Lower levels of ability are also inferred and scored.

## The Concept of Verticality

When Piaget and Inhelder (1967) asked 5-year-olds to draw trees or houses on the outline of a mountain, they drew these inside the mountain. As children matured, they drew trees and houses perpendicular to the slope; and as they reached the age of 8 or 9, began to draw them upright.

To determine whether respondents have acquired the concept of verticality, the third task, Predictive Drawing, presents the drawing of a house on top of a steep mountain and asks respondents to draw the way the house would appear if moved to a spot marked $X$ on the slope. The task is based on the premise that a respondent who draws a vertical house that is cantilevered or supported by posts has acquired the concept of verticality (5 points), and that lower levels of development can be inferred and scored.

# Drawing from Observation

There is sound reason behind the cartoon cliché of an artist squinting along the brush he holds upright at the end of his outstretched arm. Art students were taught to do just that because it is a time-honored way to assess horizontality and verticality, and compare lengths and widths, as well as angles and other spatial relationships.

In tracing the development of spatial concepts, Piaget and Inhelder (1967) have noted that young children tend to regard objects in isolation, their various features perceived in turn. Gradually, children begin to regard objects in relation to nearby objects, linking them into a single system by coordinating different points of view. At the same time, they begin to develop the idea of straight lines, parallels, and angles. Eventually, children arrive at a system embracing objects in three dimensions: left/right (horizontal relationships), above/below (vertical relationships), and front/back (relationships in depth).

The aim of the SDT Drawing from Observation task is to find out whether a respondent has acquired the ability to represent height, width, and depth, as well as assess the level of ability at the time the task is presented. It presents four simple objects arranged in a predetermined way on a straight-sided sheet of paper below eye level so that the surface of the paper is viewed as a flat plane rather than a line. The objects include three cylinders differing in height and width and a small stone. Respondents are asked to draw what they see. Scoring is based on ability to represent spatial relationships in height, width, and depth.

## Children, Adolescents, and Adults with Disabilities

The principal aim of my doctoral dissertation was to find out whether studio art experiences provided opportunities to enhance the conceptual thinking, adjustment, and aptitudes of children who had hearing impairments and language deficiencies (Silver, 1966, 1978, 2000a). In addition, I hoped to challenge the claim that the artwork of children who are deaf is inferior to the artwork of hearing children, in both subject matter and technique. With this in mind, I asked two panels of judges to evaluate the artwork produced by my students in four schools for deaf children.

One panel included 20 psychologists; psychiatrists; teachers of special education; and educators of deaf, aphasic, and hearing children. The judges attended an exhibition of drawings and paintings by my students and responded to a questionnaire, which asked whether they found evidence that art experiences provided opportunities for various kinds of cognition and evidence that would be useful in assessing various characteristics and needs. Of their 337 answers, 315 (93%) were positive, 8 (2%) were negative, and 14 (5%) were qualified.

Judging the same paintings and drawings, the second panel of 20 art educators was asked if they found evidence of spontaneity, planning, storytelling, sensitivity, and skill. Of their 260 answers, 243 (93%) were positive, 1 was negative, and 16 were qualified.

The project's findings seemed to support five concluding observations—among them, that drawing and painting could serve as instruments for expressing thoughts and feelings that cannot be verbalized and as instruments for assessing abilities, knowledge, interests, attitudes, and needs. The findings also suggested that art symbols could serve as instruments for organizing thoughts and experiences and developing ability to recall, generalize, evaluate, and imagine.

Subsequently, I received a grant from the U.S. Office of Education to conduct a demonstration project in art education for adults, as well as children, with hearing impairments.

## A Demonstration Project for Children and Adults with Hearing Impairments

The principal aim of this project was to collect information about aptitudes, interests, and vocational opportunities in the visual arts for children and adults with hearing impairments (Silver, 1967). Although the board of directors of the New York Society for the Deaf had sponsored the project, its administrators had doubts. One warned that those who came to my art class would expect to be paid for their trouble; another warned that my biggest problem would be getting a population to work with. They were mistaken. We were overwhelmed with applications as soon as it was announced that free art classes and visits to museums were available, and 54 children and adults attended the program's two semesters. They were not selected but were accepted in the order in which they applied.

After several months of weekly art classes, 12 children and one adult volunteered to take the figural form of the Torrance Test of Creative Thinking, a test of creativity in general. Their average scores were in the 99th percentile in both originality and elaboration, in the 97th percentile in fluency, and the 88th percentile in flexibility.

As in the doctoral project, panels of judges evaluated the artwork produced. In one of five assessments, three art educators judged paintings by 22 hearing students and 22 students with hearing impairments, based on originality, expressiveness, and sensitivity. The 44 paintings were identified only by number and by the age of the painter. Mean scores of the hearing-impaired children and adults were slightly higher than mean scores of hearing children and adults, whereas the mean score of hearing-impaired adolescents was slightly lower. The other assessments found that the scores of students with hearing impairments were equal or superior to scores of their hearing counterparts.

When the project ended, the adults formed an art club to continue visiting museums together. Some of its members began to correspond with me in 1970, and have continued into 2006. Three had professional careers in the visual arts. One received a bachelor of fine arts degree and continues to teach sculpture to hearing adults; another was given exhibitions of his paintings by a New York City gallery; and the third returned to his home in India, where he began to arrange for annual exhibitions of artwork by deaf children and adults not only in India but also elsewhere in Asia. I have given our correspondences to the archives of Gallaudet University.

## Two Smithsonian Institution Traveling Exhibitions

### Shout in Silence

Beginning in 1969, the Smithsonian Institution circulated an exhibition of drawings and paintings by these adults and my students in previous art classes. Explanatory texts accompanied their drawings and paintings to show that the visual arts can be especially helpful in the education of students with hearing impairments, providing opportunities for abstract thinking, imaginary play, and expressing thoughts and feelings that cannot be verbalized. A second aim was to demonstrate that these children and adults have aptitudes, interests, and vocational opportunities that are largely unexplored. The exhibition was shown at art centers around the country and extended several times until 1976.

Thereafter, the Metropolitan Museum of Art in New York showed the exhibition. It also published a catalog (Silver, 1976a) and invited the exhibitors to an opening reception. We had a grand reunion and agreed to continue the exhibition elsewhere. Its second tour began at the Kennedy Center for the Performing Arts in Washington, DC, and continued until 1987 when it was donated to the Junior Arts Center Museum in Los Angeles, together with a second exhibition circulated by the Smithsonian Institution, *Art as Language for the Handicapped* (Silver, 1979), which presented art procedures for developing and testing cognitive skills.

## Art as Language

The second exhibition included drawings and paintings by adult stroke patients as well as students with learning disabilities or language impairments. It presented their responses to drawing tasks designed to teach and test the understanding of three concepts: space, sequential order, and class inclusion. This exhibition was circulated from 1979 to 1983 in 16 states around the country.

# The State Urban Education Project

To continue investigating cognitive skills, I applied for a grant from the New York State Department of Education to conduct a state urban education project (Silver, 1973). Approval of the project arrived late, after the 1972 school year had started in September. Because my project proposal called for pretests in October and a project evaluator had not yet been assigned, I was obliged to improvise the pretest myself. A specialist at a nearby university helped me design the required 30-item criterion referenced test in exchange for one of my paintings. The pre-and posttests included rating scales for assessing ability to sequence, predict, conserve, select, combine, and represent spatial concepts as well as thoughts and feelings.

The project had three objectives: (1) to help an experimental group of children with impairments acquire concepts basic in reading and mathematics; (2) to devise procedures for developing the concepts through art experiences; and (3) to devise tasks for assessing the procedures. The project was conducted in a school for children with language and hearing impairments. It included experimental and control groups selected at random and compared these children with children who had no known impairments.

The project was also concerned with reconciling different views. Some educators had claimed that children who are deaf lack aptitude for art. Some art therapists believed that structuring art experience inhibits spontaneity, and some art educators believed that using art for therapeutic purposes interferes with aesthetic development. I hoped the project would demonstrate that therapeutic and aesthetic goals need not conflict, that art experiences can be structured without sacrificing spontaneity, and that we can pursue therapeutic and cognitive goals without neglecting aesthetic goals.

The children with language impairments had receptive and expressive language disorders. Some children had both, and most had peripheral hearing loss as well.

The experimental group of 34 children included a randomly selected 50% sample of 12 classes in the school. They attended weekly 40-minute art classes for 11 weeks in the fall and 9 weeks in the spring. The remaining 34 children, who did not participate in an art program, served as the control group. Their ages ranged from 8 to 15 years.

Drawing tasks were developed and administered as pre- and posttests for the fall program in September and January and for the spring program in January and June. The tests also were administered (once) to 68 unimpaired children in a suburban public school in order to compare groups that had and did not have impairments.

The developmental procedures emphasized exploratory learning to encourage reflection and elicit spontaneous responses. They were designed to establish an atmosphere in which independence and initiative would be self-rewarding. The procedures consisted primarily of open-ended drawing and painting tasks; when they couldn't be open-ended, they were followed by free-choice art activities. The drawing tasks focused on sequencing and relating subjects to one another, and were designed to help students detect similarities and combine subjects based on form, content, or both. For example, the children were shown two arrays of stimulus drawings—people and animals on one table, passive animals and things on another—then asked to select subjects from both tables to use in some way in their own storytelling drawings. I structured the first two classes this way to encourage the children to select, combine, and represent. Thereafter, most selected their subject matter spontaneously, without stimulus drawings.

The sequencing tasks were meant to develop concepts of space through observation and manipulation. In one task, objects on a sheet of paper served as points of reference, with the paper's edges as frames of reference. For example, I placed a cylinder and two building blocks on a sheet of paper and traced their outlines with a pencil, then asked students to select the same objects, arrange them the same way, and trace their outlines. When the drawings were superimposed and held up to a light, the children examined the outlines, noting overlaps and distances.

To develop sequencing abilities, I presented a series of cards in one color but in progressively paler tints. Asked if the colors were the same or different, the children considered similarities and differences. Then they were asked to scramble the cards and finally to place them in order from light to dark tints.

Each student received a paper palette, palette knife, and poster paints in muffin trays. After a demonstration in which paint was mixed into a series of tints, students were asked to place a dab of white in one corner of their palettes and additional colors in two other corners, then to find out how many colors they could create between them. Finally, they added black in the fourth corner and completed the circle with shades as well as tints. In the remaining time, they were free to paint as they chose. Some children painted abstract designs; others, figurative paintings (see also chapter 13).

A third task, locating a doll on a model landscape, was adapted from experiments by Piaget and Inhelder (1967, p. 421). Two identical landscapes were constructed on cafeteria trays—mountains, rivers, paths, trees, houses, and dolls made from plaster, cardboard, matchsticks, and clay. To play the game, children had to place their dolls in the same position as other people's dolls in the other landscape. After a few trials, one landscape was turned 180 degrees, making it necessary to relate the dolls to positions in the landscape, rather than to one's own position. The model landscapes had 17 marked positions.

To develop concepts of space, the children drew from observation. For example, several objects were placed on a table in front of the room—cylinders made from rolls of construction paper and bugs made from pebbles by adding legs and eyes. The arrangement was presented on a drawing board, with another board, supported by the wall, serving as backdrop. After demonstrating with a quick sketch of the arrangement, I asked the children to sketch it, then moved the arrangement to the center of the room surrounded by the children's desks. The children were asked to sketch the arrangement from at least three points of view. From one desk, the bug appeared to the left of a blue cylinder and from the opposite desk, to the right.

The project also included in-service workshops for classroom teachers. We met weekly for an hour to discuss objectives and methods, and when the first term ended, the teachers scored the posttests and the second term pre- and posttests, which included 14 items adapted from tasks in the art program.

When pre- and posttest scores of experimental and control groups in the fall program were compared, significant differences in favor of the experimental group were found. Subsequent analysis by John Kleinhans, PhD, also found significant improvement.

The median score for experimental and control groups combined was 9.37. The median of the experimental group was 11.75; of the control group, 8.5. Of the 18 experimental students, 14 had scores exceeding the combined median and 4 fell below; of the 18 control students, 3 were above and 15 below the combined median.

The chi-square value derived from the resulting 2 × 2 contingency table was 11.15. The observed chi square exceeded the criterion value of 10.83 required for the rejection of the null hypothesis of no difference between the groups at the .001 level of confidence. Thus, the observed difference between groups in favor of the experimental group was shown to be highly significant.

## The Drawing from Imagination Subtest

In a comparison of mean pre- and posttest scores of the impaired experimental group ($n = 34$, fall and spring programs combined), significant improvement was found after the art programs (pretest mean = 8.0; posttest mean = 11.47; $t = 3.62$, significant at the .01 level with 33 df [two-tailed test]). For the control group ($n = 16$) no significant difference was found (pretest mean = 8.18; posttest mean = 8.44).

In a comparison of groups with and without impairments, no significant difference was found on the pretest, but on the posttest, significant difference was found at the .05 level in favor of the experimental group with impairments. These responses are shown in figures 6.1 and 6.2.

## The Drawing from Observation Subtest

In a comparison of mean pre-and posttest scores of the impaired experimental group in the spring program ($n = 16$; teaching and testing procedures were developed during the fall program), significant improvement was found after the art program (pretest mean = 9.37; posttest mean = 11.43, $t = 3.03$, significant at the .05 level with 15 df [two-tailed test]). For the control group ($n = 16$), no significant difference was found (pretest mean = 8.56; posttest mean = 8.50).

In a comparison of groups with and without impairments, no significant difference was found.

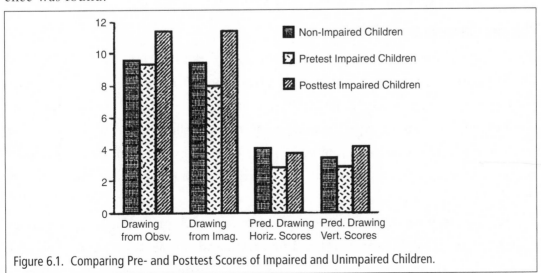

Figure 6.1. Comparing Pre- and Posttest Scores of Impaired and Unimpaired Children.

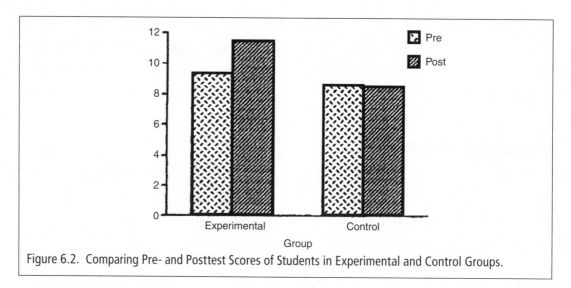

Figure 6.2. Comparing Pre- and Posttest Scores of Students in Experimental and Control Groups.

### The Predictive Drawing Subtest

In a comparison of mean pre-and posttest scores of the experimental groups with impairments (fall and spring programs combined, $n = 34$), significant improvement was found after the art programs (pretest mean in horizontal orientation = 2.88; posttest mean = 3.76, $t = 5.50$, significant at the .01 level with 67 df; pretest mean in vertical orientation = 2.91; posttest mean = 4.11; $t = 8.57$, significant at the .01 level).

### Comparing the 68 Unimpaired Children with Both Groups of Children with Impairments

Significant differences were found on the pretest in favor of the unimpaired group. On the posttest, no significant difference was found in vertical orientation, but significant difference was found in horizontal orientation at the .05 level of probability in favor of the experimental group with impairments.

### Changes in Creativity and Art Skills

To test the theory that emphasizing cognition need not interfere with aesthetic and creative growth, two judges—a university professor of art and a registered art therapist/painter—were asked to evaluate three drawings or paintings produced by each child in the fall program experimental group ($n = 18$): the child's first work, the last work, and a work produced at midterm. The 54 drawings and paintings were identified only by number and shown in random order to conceal the sequence in which they had been produced.

The judges, working independently, rated each work on a scale of 1 to 5 points for sensitivity and skill, as well as for ability to represent objects or events. The scale ranged from the low level (imitative, learned, impersonal, 1 point), to a moderate level (going beyond description to elaborate or edit an experience, 3 points), to the high level (beyond restructuring, highly personal, imaginative, inventive, 5 points).

Both judges found improvements that were significant at the .01 level. As rated by the art therapist/painter, the mean score for artwork produced in the first class was 4.44; the mean score for work produced in the last class was 7.27 ($t = 3.13$, significant at the $p < 0.01$ level). As rated by the university professor of art, the mean score of the work produced in the first class was 3.66, and the last class, 6.33 ($t = 3.29$, significant at the $p < 0.01$ level).

In skill and expressiveness combined, the university professor of art gave four children the lowest score on their first works and the highest score on their last works. The art therapist/painter found the same improvements in six children (Silver, 1973; 1978; 1986; 1989b, p. 225).

Thus, the findings of this study support the theory that emphasizing cognitive development need not interfere with aesthetic and creative development. The study found evidence of pretest-posttest gains in both cognitive and creative skills before and after the 11-week art therapy program, evidence that cognitive, aesthetic, and therapeutic goals can be pursued concurrently.

The study also found evidence of initial cognitive differences between children with language/hearing impairments and children with no known impairments, as well as evidence that art therapy interventions seem to bring about change, enabling the group with impairments to catch up and even excel. Before the art program, the children in the experimental group lagged behind in the Drawing from Imagination and Predictive Drawing tasks. After the art program, they equaled or surpassed the unimpaired children.

Subsequently, between 1974 and 1982, the SDT rating scales and developmental tasks were refined and amended in working with additional clinical and nonclinical populations, as will be discussed in chapter 10.

## Children with Visual Motor Disorders

In a second study, we asked whether the teaching and testing procedures would be useful with children who had an opposite constellation of skills—verbal strengths and visual-motor weaknesses—and whether the procedures could be used effectively by therapists other than the one who developed them (Silver & Lavin, 1977).

Those who participated were 11 graduate students who had registered for an elective course in art therapy, working individually, under supervision, with 11 unselected children with learning disabilities. The art program consisted of 10 weekly one-hour sessions. This study used the procedures used previously in the state urban education project to determine whether the developmental and assessment procedures were effective. This study did not have a control group.

The children who participated were not selected. Announcements were sent to newspapers and to the Westchester County, New York, Association for Children with Learning Disabilities, stating that art classes were being offered to these children at the College of New Rochelle. The first 15 children who applied were enrolled. One child had been diagnosed as hyperkinetic. Another was severely disturbed and attended a day school in a psychiatric hospital. The others attended private schools or special classes in public schools. All but two had disabilities of a visual-spatial motor nature, and these two were eliminated from the statistical analysis. Also eliminated were children who withdrew or whose art therapist became ill, leaving 11 children in the study. The classes were held on Saturday mornings, with all participants working in a large studio under my supervision.

The art program provided frequent opportunities to associate and reflect; draw from observation and from different points of view; model clay; mix poster paints into sequences of color; and select and combine colors, shapes, and subject matter while drawing or painting from imagination. Emphasis was on content rather than on form, on meaningful pictures rather than on abstract designs, on exploratory learning rather than on directive teaching, and on eliciting responses rather than on instructing. Other procedures did not involve drawing, such as placing cylinders in order on a matrix. The children's first and last drawings from imagination were assessed for ability to select, combine, and represent.

## Results

Claire Lavin, PhD, analyzed the results using an analysis of variance to determine interscorer reliability. She found coefficients of .852 in ability to select and combine, and .944 in spatial orientation, as is reported in chapter 8. She evaluated the effectiveness of the training program by using a $t$ test ($n = 11$) for correlated means to determine the significance of differences in mean pre- and posttest scores and performed separate analyses for scores on the tests of ability to form groups (select and combine), spatial orientation, and ability to order a matrix. All the obtained $t$ values were statistically significant. Improvements in ability to form groups ($t = 4.79$) and in ordering a matrix ($t = 6.54$) were significant at the .01 level. Improvement in spatial orientation was significant at the .05 level ($t = 2.42$). Thus, the children with learning disabilities who participated in the therapeutic program improved significantly in the three areas of cognitive development that were the focus of the study.

The success of this training program seems to indicate that cognitively oriented art experiences can be used to help children with learning disabilities express concepts nonverbally, through visual–motor channels, in spite of impaired functioning in this area.

Three years after the project ended, four of the graduate students had become registered art therapists who were coauthors of the study that follows.

## National Institute of Education Project for Children Performing below Grade Level

In 1979, I received a grant from the National Institute of Education to conduct a project designed to verify previous results with a wider variety of setting and more diverse populations (Silver et al., 1980). It also examined relationships between the SDT and traditional, language-oriented measures of intelligence or achievement.

The 84 children who participated had been nominated by school administrators, based on performing at least one year below grade level in reading or mathematics. They ranged in age from 7 to 11 and attended five schools: a private school for learning disabled children, and four public schools, which provided classes for children with special needs.

As originally planned, the experimental group would include only children who scored at least 3 points in the Drawing from Imagination task. As it happened, however, we had to include children with lower scores in order to have 20 children in each school, 10 in the experimental group participating in the art program, and 10 in the control group receiving no special treatment. The selected children were randomly assigned to experimental and control groups. During the art program, several children were lost for various reasons, and additional children were randomly removed to equate the number in each group for statistical analysis.

In each school, an art therapist worked with two groups of five children each for approximately 40 minutes a week for 12 weeks. During the first six weeks, all art therapists used the same art procedures. During the second six weeks, they adapted the procedures to meet the needs of individual children, and devised procedures of their own.

Before and after the art program, the children in both experimental and control groups were given the SDT, the Otis-Lennon School Ability Test, and the Metropolitan Reading and Arithmetic Test. Because some were too severely impaired to take the Otis-Lennon and Metropolitan Tests, their school records were used instead. In addition, art therapists and teachers elsewhere had volunteered to give the SDT to other students and send us the test booklets to score, as well as the children's scores on traditional tests of intelligence and achievement. These scores were correlated and analyzed to determine the relationship of the SDT to these measures. The findings are included among studies of reliability and validity in chapter 8.

The developmental procedures included drawing, painting, modeling clay, and playing the manipulative "games" designed in the state urban education project for developing conceptual, sequential, and spatial skills. The procedures are presented in detail elsewhere (Silver, 1996c, 2000a, 2001).

To determine the effectiveness of the programs, Claire Lavin, PhD, examined the significance of differences between the pre- and posttest scores of experimental and control subjects, using an analysis of variance for repeated measures. The experimental group improved significantly in total scores between the pre- and posttests. The gains made by the experimental group were higher than those made by the control group, but not significantly higher.

A similar procedure was performed with respect to gains in general intelligence as measured by the Otis-Lennon test. The experimental group failed to demonstrate significantly higher posttest scores than control subjects.

The final objective program was to determine whether children in a specific setting made significantly greater gains than children in different settings. A school-by-school analysis was conducted for each variable, using a series of tests.

In general, the SDT scores of experimental subjects tended to be higher than those of control group subjects. Only in three instances, however, were these differences statistically significant. In one school (the school for children with learning disabilities) both the total SDT score and the Drawing from Imagination score were significantly higher for experimental subjects. In another school, the experimental children scored significantly higher in the Drawing from Observation task.

The project report also included a case study by each art therapist, providing qualitative as well as quantitative information. Although the gains made by some children were not reflected in their posttest scores, gains became evident in classroom behavior.

## Discussion

In the state urban education project and the previous study, we found significant gains in cognitive skills within a similar time period. In the National Institute of Education Project, the experimental group again improved significantly. Although their gains were higher than control group gains, they were not significantly higher. It may be that the procedures must be extended beyond 12 sessions if a differential impact is to be observed. Another factor that may have affected the findings is that the children in this study were a more heterogeneous group than those studied previously. Many of the children nominated by school administrators were slow learners, not language-impaired. It may be that these children have a generalized low functioning and do not benefit from art experiences. It had been our intention to select children with high scores on the SDT. The limited number of children with this pattern required us to select children not as strong as initially planned.

It is not clear why the school for children with learning disabilities was the only school with significant differences between posttest scores of experimental and control groups, nor why the gains in the previous studies failed to materialize. The finding may reflect the superior skills of one art therapist, the different constellations of strengths and weaknesses among children with learning disabilities, or too much flexibility in the art program. By specifying what procedures to use in only 6 of the 12 sessions, we may have introduced too many variables.

The results of the testing program indicate that there is a relationship between the SDT and other tests of intelligence and achievement. Although moderate, it nevertheless indicates that the SDT is measuring cognitive skills. As such, the SDT can serve as an instrument for identifying children who have cognitive skills that escape detection on traditional tests. The skills involved in the Drawing from Imagination and Predictive Drawing tasks are similar to the skills required in reading, math, and traditional tests. That also explains why some children do well on the SDT although they do not do well on traditional measures; we are using a different medium to tap these cognitive skills. In 1983, the SDT was published by Special Child Publications; revised editions were published in 1990, 1996, and 2002.

# Chapter 7

# Administering and Scoring the Silver Drawing Test

◇     ◇     ◇

This chapter includes guidelines for administering the Silver Drawing Test (SDT) and scoring responses to the three drawing tasks as well as examples of scored responses. The test booklet, scoring forms, and other test materials may be found in appendix A.

The SDT has been administered and scored without prior training by teachers as well as by mental health professionals in America, Australia, Brazil, Russia, and Thailand, as will be discussed in chapter 12. The recommended age range is from five years to adult. Individual administration is suggested for children younger than seven and for clinical subjects.

The SDT is not timed, but usually takes about 15 minutes. Although each of the three tasks can be considered separately and is scored separately, they are interconnected and begin with the simplest task, Predictive Drawing. It asks the respondent to predict changes in the appearance of objects by adding lines to outline drawings. The second task, Drawing from Observation, asks the respondent to draw an arrangement of three cylinders and a large pebble to assess ability to represent spatial relationships in height, width, and depth. Both tasks are usually completed in about five minutes.

## The Silver Drawing Test and Draw a Story

The third task, Drawing from Imagination, aims to stimulate reflection and usually takes about 10 minutes. It is important to prevent interruptions or distractions, particularly because some respondents become deeply absorbed in modifying and elaborating their drawings (or stories). For this reason, I recommend pencils with erasers rather than pens, markers, or crayons.

It is also important to establish an atmosphere that is encouraging and supportive. As an introduction, say:

> I believe you will have fun with this kind of drawing. You will be asked to draw things you can see, things you cannot see, and things only you can imagine. It doesn't matter whether or not you have talent in drawing. What matters is using your imagination and expressing your own ideas.

As much as possible, avoid the stress usually associated with testing. Accommodate reasonable requests and encourage questions before drawing begins. After it has begun, prevent interruptions and postpone discussions as much as possible until all respondents have finished. Provide a test booklet for yourself as well as for each respondent.

## The Predictive Drawing Task

The Predictive Drawing Task is shown in figure 7.1. If a respondent has difficulty reading directions, use pantomime or manual language. For example, hold up your own booklet, point to the first glass on the left, and say, "Here is an ice cream soda. Suppose you drank a few sips." Then draw a horizontal line near the top of your second glass and say, "Can you draw lines in the glasses to show how the soda would look if you took a few sips, then a few more, and more, until you gradually drank it all?"

You also might pantomime with a drinking straw, taking care not to make a sequence of gestures or indicate where the lines should be drawn. If you use manual language, modify the directions as needed.

Guidelines for scoring responses are shown in table 7.1, and examples of scored responses in figures 7.2 to 7.8.

Suppose you took a few sips of a soda, then a few more, and more, until your glass was empty. Can you draw lines in the glasses to show how the soda would look if you gradually drank it all?

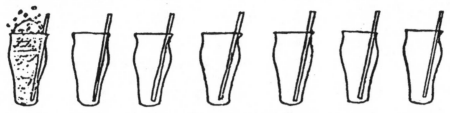

Suppose you tilted a bottle half filled with water. Can you draw lines in the bottles to show how the water would look?

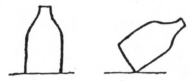

Suppose you put the house on the spot marked x. Can you draw the way it would look?

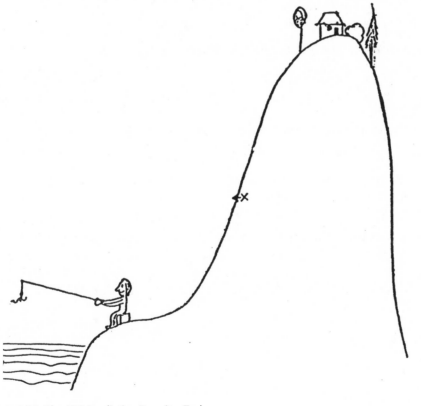

Figure 7.1. The SDT Predictive Drawing Task.

© 1983–2007 by Rawley Silver. Reprinted with permission for personal use only.

---

### Table 7.1 Guidelines for Scoring the Predictive Drawing Task of the SDT

---

**Predicting a Sequence**

| | |
|---|---|
| 0 points | No sequence representing the soda in the glasses |
| 1 point | Incomplete sequence |
| 2 points | Two or more sequences |
| 3 points | Descending series of lines with corrections (trial and error) |
| 4 points | A sequence with unevenly spaced increments but no corrections |
| 5 points | A sequence with evenly spaced increments and no corrections (systematic) |

*Note:* The sequence does not have to continue to the bottom of the glass

**Predicting Horizontality***

| | |
|---|---|
| 0 points | No line representing water surface is inside the tilted bottle |
| 1 point | Line parallels bottom or sides of tilted bottle (suggesting that the frame of reference is inside the bottle) |
| 2 points | Line almost parallels bottom or side of tilted bottle |
| 3 points | Line is oblique (suggesting that the frame of reference is external but not related to the table surface) |
| 4 points | Line seems related to the table surface but is not parallel |
| 5 points | Line is parallel to table surface within 5 degrees |

**Predicting Verticality***

| | |
|---|---|
| 0 points | No representation of the house or, if examinee is younger than five years, the house is inside the mountain |
| 1 point | House is approximately perpendicular to the slope. |
| 2 points | House is neither perpendicular nor vertical, but on a slant or upside down |
| 3 points | House is vertical but has inadequate support; may be entirely inside the mountain if examinee is older than five years |
| 4 points | House is vertical but has inadequate support, such as partly inside the mountain |
| 5 points | House is vertical, supported by posts, columns, platforms, or other structures |

---

*Note:* The tasks for predicting horizontality and verticality are adapted from experiments by Piaget and Inhelder (1967).

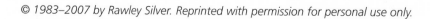

© 1983–2007 by Rawley Silver. Reprinted with permission for personal use only.

## Examples of Scored Responses to the Predictive Drawing Task

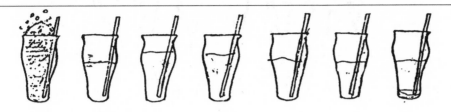

0 points: No sequence representing the soda in the glasses.

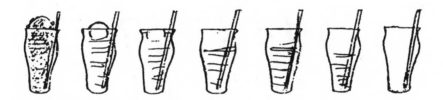

1 point: Incomplete sequence.

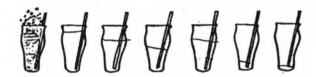

2 points: Two or more sequences.

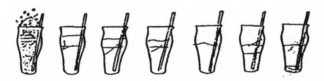

3 points: Descending series of lines with corrections (trial and error).

Figure 7.2. Predicting a Sequence.

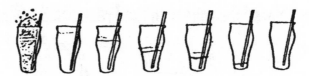

3 points: Descending series of lines with corrections.

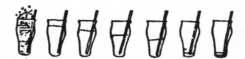

4 points: Sequence with unevenly spaced increments but no corrections.

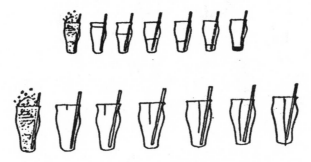

5. Sequence with evenly spaced increments and no corrections (systematic).

Figure 7.2.  continued

1 point: Line parallels bottom or side of tilted bottle.

2 points: Line almost parallels bottom or sides.

3 points: Line is oblique.

4 points: Line relates to the table surface but is not quite parallel.

5 points: Line is parallel to the table surface within 5 degrees.

Figure 7.3. Predicting Horizontality.

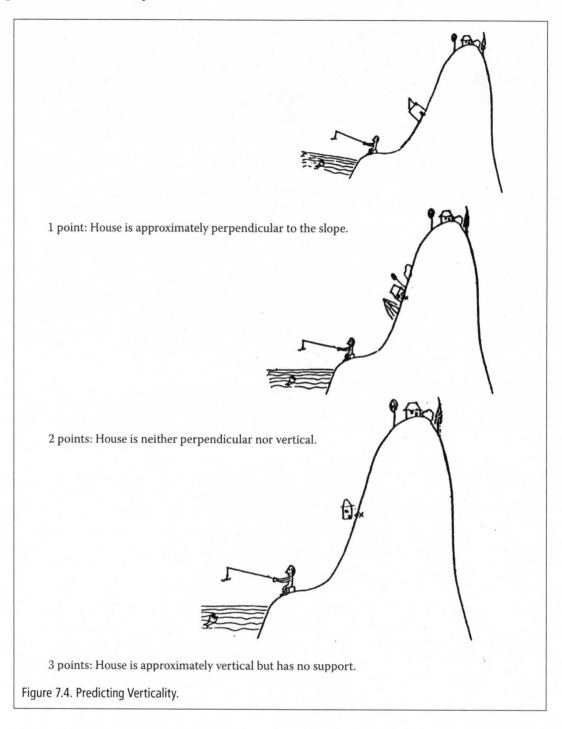

1 point: House is approximately perpendicular to the slope.

2 points: House is neither perpendicular nor vertical.

3 points: House is approximately vertical but has no support.

Figure 7.4. Predicting Verticality.

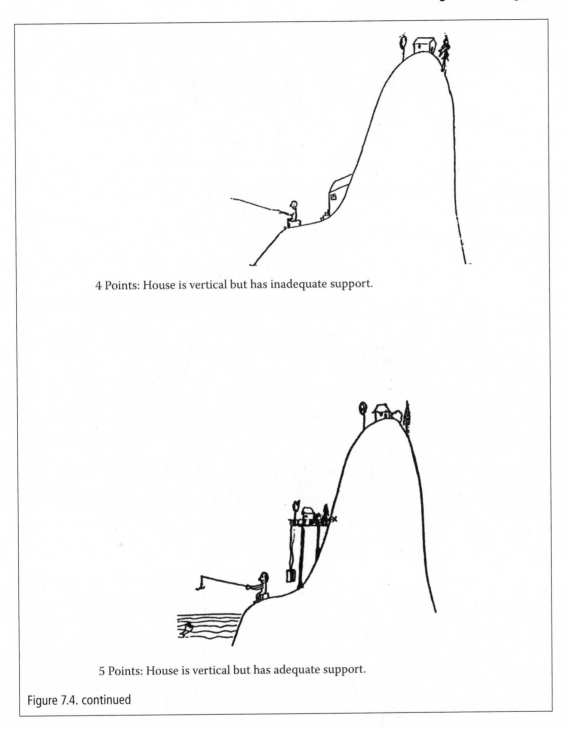

4 Points: House is vertical but has inadequate support.

5 Points: House is vertical but has adequate support.

Figure 7.4. continued

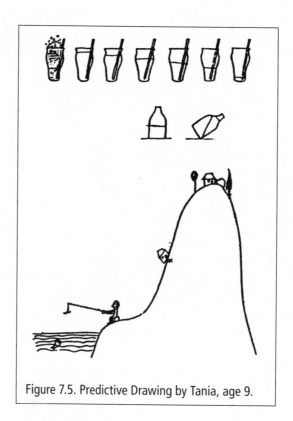

Figure 7.5. Predictive Drawing by Tania, age 9.

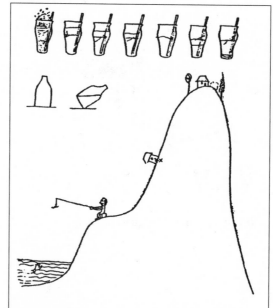

Figure 7.6. Predictive Drawing by an Adult in a University Audience.

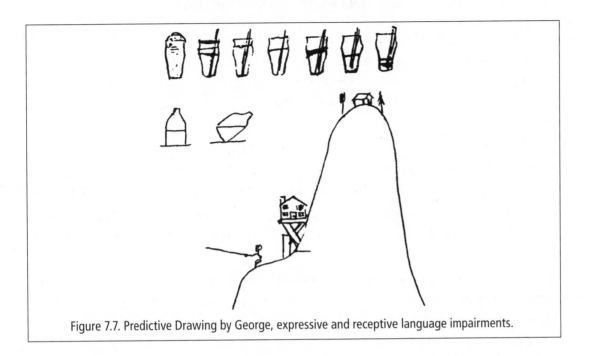

Figure 7.7. Predictive Drawing by George, expressive and receptive language impairments.

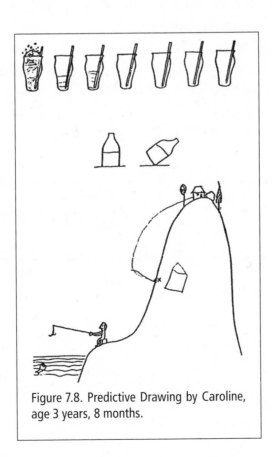

Figure 7.8. Predictive Drawing by Caroline, age 3 years, 8 months.

# The Drawing from Observation Task

Prepare the arrangement in advance, placing the layout sheet on a table below eye level so that it will appear as a plane rather than as a line (if placed above eye level, it will appear as a line, preventing perception of depth); then place the cylinders and a large pebble or stone on their outlines on the layout sheet. The arrangement should appear as sketched in the guidelines for scoring (see table 7.2)—that is, the widest cylinder appears on the left, the tallest on the right, and the smallest to the left of the stone between them.

If the task is to be administered to groups, long, narrow tables are useful. An arrangement can be placed at both ends, with chairs along both sides of the tables. Check the viewpoint from the farthest seats so that no one sits too far to the left or right of the arrangement.

If a respondent has difficulty reading directions, hold up your booklet at the drawing page shown in figure 7.10, pantomime sketching the arrangement (for no more than five seconds), then read aloud the directions:

"Have you ever tried to draw something just the way it looks? Here are some things to draw. Look at them carefully, then draw what you see in the space below."

Sketches of the arrangement are shown below. The front view can serve as the criterion for drawings scored 5 points.

When scoring, note that cylinder #1 (on the left) should be the widest and #4 (on the right) should be is the tallest; cylinder #2 should be in the foreground; and the stone #3, is behind and between #2 and #4. To examinees seated toward the left, #2 will appear farther from #1 and closer to #3. To examinees seated toward the right, #2 will appear farther from #3 and closer to #1.

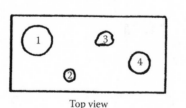

Top view

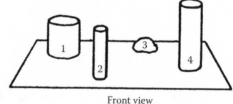

Front view

### Table 7.2  Guidelines for Scoring the Drawing from Observation Task of the SDT

Horizontal (Left/Right) Relationships

| | |
|---|---|
| 0 points | Horizontal relationships are confused; no objects are in the correct left-right order |
| 1 point | Only one object is in the correct left-right order |
| 2 points | Two objects are in the correct left-right order |
| 3 points | Three adjacent objects or two pairs of objects are in the correct left-right order. |
| 4 points | All four objects are approximately correct in order but not carefully observed or represented |
| 5 points | All objects are in the correct left-right order |

Vertical (Above/Below) Relationships (Height)

| | |
|---|---|
| 0 points | All objects are flat; no representation of height |
| 1 point | All objects are about the same height |
| 2 points | Two objects (not necessarily adjacent) are approximately correct in height |
| 3 points | Three objects (not necessarily adjacent) are approximately correct in height |
| 4 points | All four objects are approximately correct in height but are not carefully observed and represented |
| 5 points | All vertical relationships are represented accurately |

Front/Back Relationships (Depth)

| | |
|---|---|
| 0 points | All objects are in a horizontal row even though arrangement was presented below eye level, or no adjacent objects are correctly related in depth |
| 1 point | One object is above or below a baseline (drawn or implied), or front-back relationships are incorrect |
| 2 points | Two objects (not necessarily adjacent) are approximately correct in front-back relationships |
| 3 points | Three adjacent objects or two pairs of objects are approximately correct in front-back relationships |
| 4 points | All four objects are approximately correct in front-back relationships but not well observed and represented |
| 5 points | All front-back relationships are represented accurately and the layout sheet is included in the drawing |

© 1983–2007 by Rawley Silver. Reprinted with permission for personal use only.

# The Silver Drawing Test and Draw a Story

Have you ever tried to draw something just the way it looks? Here are some things to draw. Look at them carefully, then draw what you see in the space below.

Figure 7.9. The SDT Drawing from Observation Task.

## Examples of Scored Responses to the Drawing from Observation Task

Horizontal relationships: 4 points. (All four objects are approximately correct in left-right order but not carefully observed and represented.)

Vertical relationships: 4 points. (All four objects are approximately correct in height but not carefully observed and represented.)

Relationships in depth: 1 point. (One object is above the base line.)

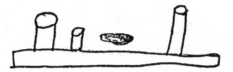

Horizontal relationships: 5 points. (The horizontal relationships are accurate.)

Vertical relationships: 5 points. (The vertical relationships are accurate.)

Relationships in depth: 5 points. (The relationships in depth are accurate and the layout sheet is included in the drawing.)

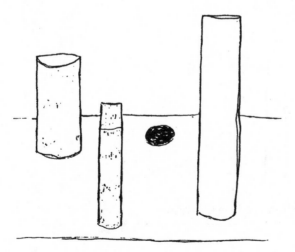

Figure 7.10. Example of Drawing from Observation.

Horizontal relationships: 0 points. (No objects are in the correct left-right order.)
Vertical relationships: 4 points. (All four objects are approximately correct in height.)
Relationships in depth: 0 points. (All objects are in a horizontal row.)

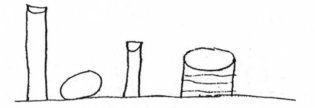

Horizontal relationships: 2 points. (Two objects are approximately correct in left-right corner.)
Vertical relationships: 3 points. (Three objects are approximately correct in height.)
Relationships in depth: 1 point. (Relationships in depth are incorrect.)

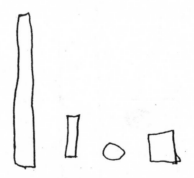

Figure 7.11. Example of Drawing from Observation.

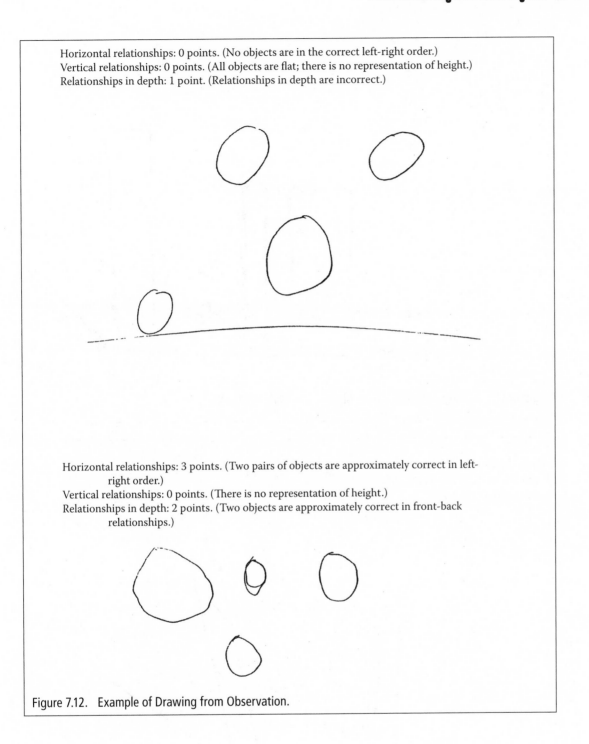

Horizontal relationships: 0 points. (No objects are in the correct left-right order.)
Vertical relationships: 0 points. (All objects are flat; there is no representation of height.)
Relationships in depth: 1 point. (Relationships in depth are incorrect.)

Horizontal relationships: 3 points. (Two pairs of objects are approximately correct in left-right order.)
Vertical relationships: 0 points. (There is no representation of height.)
Relationships in depth: 2 points. (Two objects are approximately correct in front-back relationships.)

Figure 7.12.   Example of Drawing from Observation.

| | |
|---|---|
| Left-right | 5 |
| Above-below | 5 |
| Front-back | 5 |
| Subtest Total | 15 |

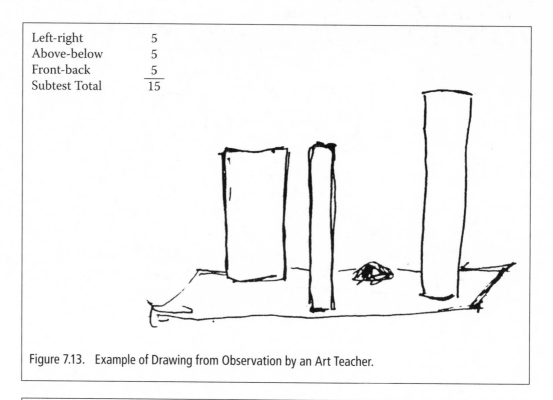

Figure 7.13.   Example of Drawing from Observation by an Art Teacher.

| | |
|---|---|
| Left-right | 2 |
| Above-below | 4 |
| Front-back | 2 |
| Subtest Total | 8 |

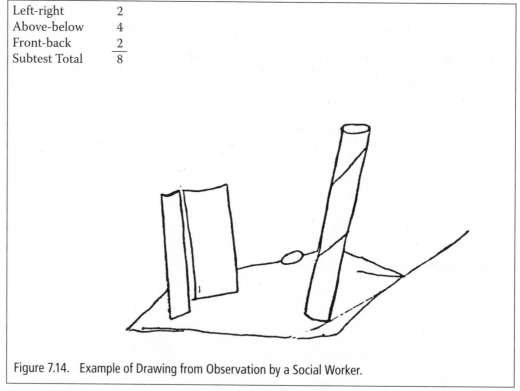

Figure 7.14.   Example of Drawing from Observation by a Social Worker.

## The Drawing from Imagination Task

If you feel respondents may have difficulty reading directions, point to the Form A set of stimulus drawings (fig. 7.15a) and the drawing page (fig. 7.16), and then say,

> Choose two picture ideas and imagine a story, something happening between the pictures you choose. When you are ready, draw a picture of what you imagine. Show what is happening in your drawing.
>
> Don't just copy these pictures. You can make changes and draw other things too.
>
> When you finish drawing, write a title or story. Tell what is happening and what may happen later on.

If a respondent chooses to draw different subjects, or simply copies the stimulus drawings, do not intervene unless you feel the instructions were misunderstood.

After the drawings are finished, ask for the information requested below the drawing. With respondents who have difficulty writing, offer to write their stories using their words.

Whenever possible, discuss the drawings individually so that meanings can be clarified. It is important to make respondents feel it is safe to express thoughts and feelings, "watched only by friends." If they used symbols or metaphors, use them, too. For example, if the principal subject is a cat, you might ask, "Can you tell me how the cat feels or what it is thinking? What has happened and what may happen later on?" Be alert for verbal clues, such as personal pronouns and the subjects of sentences. Metaphoric dialogues often provide opportunities to introduce healthier adaptations or alternative solutions.

Guidelines for scoring the cognitive content of drawings from imagination range from low to high levels of ability, scored 1 to 5 points, as presented in table 7.3. Guidelines for scoring emotional content, self-images, and humor range from strongly negative to strongly positive, also scored 1 to 5 points, as shown in tables 7.4, 7.5, and 7.6.

It is important to identify principal subjects whenever possible, and to consider what the choice of stimulus drawings suggests about those who chose them. Do the drawings reflect anger, fear, conflicts, desires, or social isolation? Are other subjects hostile or friendly?

The Form A (fig. 7.15a) set of stimulus drawings should be used only for pre- and posttesting. The second set, Form B (fig. 7.15b), is provided for any other purpose, such as developing cognitive skills or obtaining additional responses so that patterns may emerge.

# The Silver Drawing Test and Draw a Story

## Drawing What You Imagine

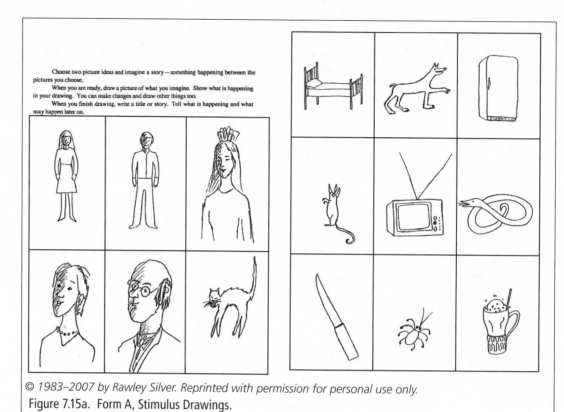

© 1983–2007 by Rawley Silver. Reprinted with permission for personal use only.

Figure 7.15a.  Form A, Stimulus Drawings.

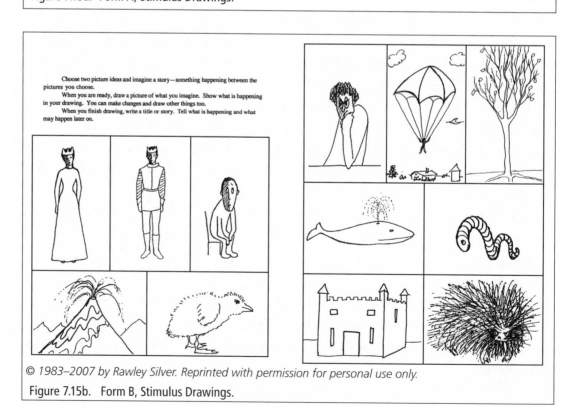

© 1983–2007 by Rawley Silver. Reprinted with permission for personal use only.

Figure 7.15b.  Form B, Stimulus Drawings.

Drawing

Story:_____

_____

_____

_____

_____

Please fill in the blanks below:

First name ____ Sex____ Age ____ Location (state): _____Date:_____

Just now I'm feeling ____very happy ____O.K. ____angry ____frightened ____sad

Figure 7.16. Drawing from Imagination Page.

---

**Table 7.3   Guidelines for Scoring the Drawing from Imagination Task of the SDT**

---

Ability to Select (Content or Meaning of the Response)

| | |
|---|---|
| 0 points | No evidence of selecting |
| 1 point | Perceptual level: single subject, or subjects unrelated in size or placement |
| 2 points | Subjects may be related in size or placement but there is no interaction |
| 3 points | Functional level: concrete, shows what subjects do, or what is done to them |
| 4 points | Descriptive rather than abstract or imaginative |
| 5 points | Conceptual level: imaginative, well-organized idea; implies more than is visible, or shows other ability to deal with abstract ideas |

Ability to Combine (The Form of the Drawing)

| | |
|---|---|
| 0 points | Single subject, no spatial relationships |
| 1 point | Proximity: subjects float in space, related only by proximity |
| 2 points | Arrows, dotted lines, or other attempts to show relationships |
| 3 points | Baseline: subjects are related to one another along a baseline (real or implied) |
| 4 points | Beyond the baseline level, but much of the drawing area is blank |
| 5 points | Overall coordination; shows depth or takes into account the entire drawing area, or else includes a series of two or more drawings |

Ability to Represent (Concepts and Creativity in the Form, Content, Title, or Story)

| | |
|---|---|
| 0 points | No evidence of representation |
| 1 point | Imitative: copies stimulus drawings or uses stick figures or stereotypes |
| 2 points | Beyond imitation, but drawing or ideas are commonplace |
| 3 points | Restructured: changes or elaborates on stimulus drawings or stereotypes |
| 4 points | Beyond restructuring: moderately original or expressive |
| 5 points | Transformational: highly original, expressive, playful, suggestive, or uses metaphors, puns, jokes, satire, or double meanings |

*© 1983–2007 by Rawley Silver. Reprinted with permission for personal use only.*

---

**Table 7.4  Scale for Assessing Emotional Content**

---

\_\_\_1   point: strongly negative emotional content; for example:

   Solitary subjects portrayed as sad, helpless, isolated, suicidal, dead, or in mortal danger

   Relationships that are destructive, murderous, or life threatening

\_\_\_2   points: moderately negative emotional content; for example:

   Solitary subjects portrayed as frightened, angry, dissatisfied, assaultive, or unfortunate

   Relationships that are stressful, hostile, destructive, or unpleasant

\_\_\_2.5 points: ambiguous or ambivalent emotional content suggesting unpleasant or unfortunate outcomes

\_\_\_3   points: neutral emotional content; for example, ambivalent, both negative and positive; unemotional, neither negative nor positive; or ambiguous or unclear

\_\_\_3.5 points: ambiguous or ambivalent emotional content suggesting hopeful, pleasant, or fortunate outcomes

\_\_\_4   points: moderately positive emotional content; for example:

   Solitary subjects portrayed as fortunate but passive, enjoying, or being rescued

   Relationships that are friendly or positive

\_\_\_5   points: strongly positive themes; for example:

   Solitary subjects portrayed as effective, happy, or achieving goals

   Relationships that are caring or loving

*© 1983–2007 by Rawley Silver. Reprinted with permission for personal use only.*

---

Table 7.5 Scale for Assessing Self-Image

___1    point: morbid fantasy; respondent seems to identify with a subject portrayed as sad, helpless, isolated, suicidal, dead, or in mortal danger

___2    points: unpleasant fantasy; respondent seems to identify with a subject portrayed as frightened, frustrated, or unfortunate

___2.5  points: unclear or ambivalent self-image with negative outcome; respondent seems to identify with a subject who appears unfortunate or likely to fail

___3    points: ambiguous or ambivalent fantasy; respondent seems to identify with a subject portrayed as ambivalent or unemotional, or else the self-image (such as the narrator) is unclear or invisible

___3.5  points: unclear, ambivalent, or negative self-image, but outcome seems positive; respondent seems to identify with a subject who appears likely to achieve goal

___4    points: pleasant fantasy; respondent seems to identify with a subject portrayed as fortunate but passive, such as being rescued

___5    points: wish-fulfilling fantasy; respondent seems to identify with a subject who is powerful, assaultive, loved, or achieving goals

*© 1983–2007 by Rawley Silver. Reprinted with permission for personal use only.*

Table 7.6 Scale for Assessing the Use of Humor (Revised)

___1    point: lethal and morbid humor; for example:
        Amused by subject(s) dying painfully or in mortal danger and overtly expressing pain and/or fear, either through words or images

___1.5  points: lethal but not morbid humor; for example:
        Amused by subject(s) disappearing, dead, or in mortal danger but not expressing pain and/or fear, either through words or images

___2    points: disparaging humor; for example:
        Amused by a principal subject who is unlike the respondent (such as of the opposite gender) and unattractive, frustrated, foolish, or unfortunate, but not in mortal danger

___2.5  points: self-disparaging humor; for example:
        Uses personal pronoun and/or is amused by a principal subject who is like the respondent as well as unattractive, frustrated, foolish, or unfortunate, but not in mortal danger

___3    points: ambiguous or ambivalent humor (neutral); for example:
        Meaning or outcome is both negative and positive, neither negative nor positive, or unclear

___4    points: resilient humor (more positive than negative); for example:
        Principal subject(s) overcomes adversity or outcome is hopeful or favorable

___5    points: playful humor (entirely positive); for example:
        Kindly, absurd, or with play on words, such as rhymes or puns

*© 1983–2007 by Rawley Silver. Reprinted with permission for personal use only.*

# Examples of Scored Responses to the Drawing from Imagination Task

## Mack

Mack is a presumably normal sixth grader in an urban public school. Presented with the Form A set of stimulus drawings, he chose the boy, the soda, and the refrigerator. In his drawing, the boy is transformed into a young athlete endowed with large biceps, broad shoulders, and tiny waist. He spreads his arms wide, holding the soda, which has been enlarged to hold two scoops of ice cream, side by side, and a striped straw that bends toward the smiling athlete. The refrigerator has also been embellished with the manufacturer's name. A fluorescent light hangs overhead and, beyond the window, the sun shines.

In emotional content, the theme of Mack's drawing is strongly positive. School has ended for the day and its solitary subject is portrayed as powerful and achieving goals. As for self-image, Mack seems to have created a wish-fulfilling fantasy and identified with his principal subject.

In ability to select, Mack's response is well organized and implies more than is visible (his subject: an athlete). Further evidence that it reflects performance at the conceptual level is the abstract word *snack* in his title, signifying a class of tasty food. In ability to combine it shows depth (the window is behind the boy), and in ability to represent, it is expressive, playful, and suggestive.

---

Emotional Content 5: principal subject seems powerful and achieving goals

Self-Image 5: Mack seems to identify (or wish to identify) with Muscleboy

Ability to Select 5: imaginative, well organized

Ability to Combine 5: overall coordination

Ability to Represent 5: expressive, playful

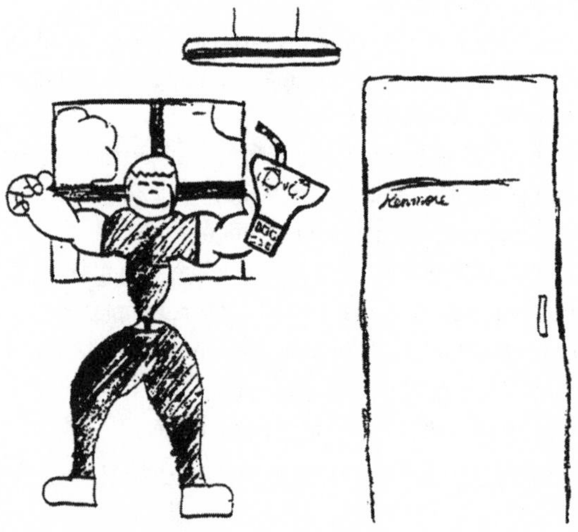

---

Figure 7.17. "Muscleboy Having a Snack after School," by Mack, age 12, no impairments.

## Dan

Dan, age 15, attended a special school for children with language impairments. His diagnosis was "congenital expressive aphasia," and he was unable to read.

Presented with the Form A set of stimulus drawings, he chose the boy, the girl, and the television. In his drawing, the boy sits on a chair watching TV, his feet resting on a footstool. Using a line to separate indoors from outdoors, the girl seems to be outside, skating on the sidewalk. At her side, but presented from a different point of view, another boy rides a bicycle.

In emotional content, Dan's theme seems moderately positive. The boy indoors is passively watching TV. The children outside are playing, but do not seem engaged in active play. In self-image, Dan may identify with one or both of the boys, but without verbal or written clues that is unclear.

In ability to select, Dan seems to have chosen his subjects at the functional level, showing what they do. In ability to combine, his use of a line to separate inside from outside suggests ability beyond the proximity level but below the baseline level. In ability to represent, Dan imitated the stimulus drawing television but drew it on a table. He also restructured the boy and girl and invented the chair, footstool, sidewalk, and bicycle.

Emotional Content 4: moderately positive
Self-Image 3: unclear
Ability to Select 3: functional; shows what subjects do
Ability to Combine 2: vertical line separates inside and outside
Ability to Represent 3: restructures stimulus drawings and adds details

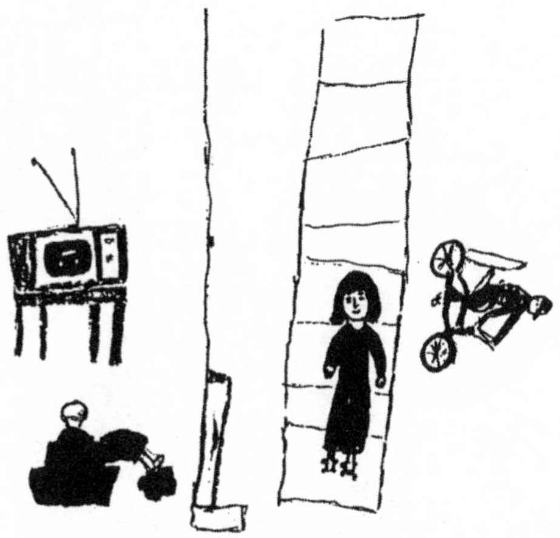

Figure 7.18.   Untitled Drawing by Dan, age 15, language impaired.

### Jody

Jody is a presumably normal girl in the fifth grade of an urban elementary school, who chose the stimulus drawing of the bride and the mouse. In her drawing, the bride is transformed. She is drawn full length and seems much younger than the stimulus drawing bride. Jody also added hands with fingers outstretched, and a gown with many details. The mouse is also transformed, holding a bouquet of flowers, and leaning toward the bride with tail held high.

In emotional content, Jody's response seems ambivalent, both negative and positive. The bride's fingers and averted gaze suggest feelings of disgust; whereas the mouse (the groom?) seems pleased. In self-image, the youthfulness of the bride suggests that Jody identifies with her.

In ability to select, this fantasy seems to be a well-organized idea, implying more than is visible, in spite of its noncommunicative title. In ability to combine, the bride seems slightly in the foreground, the mouse at a distance slightly behind her, perhaps suggesting their relative status in Jody's esteem. In ability to represent, the contradictory feelings of both bride and groom are evident.

---

Emotional Content 2.5: ambivalent, sugesting unpleasant outcome

Self-Image 2: Jody seems to identify with the disgusted bride

Ability to Select 5: implies more than is visible

Ability to Combine 4: beyond the baseline level

Ability to Represent 5: highly expressive

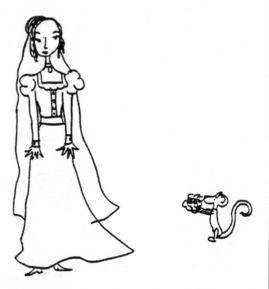

Figure 7.19. "The Bride and the Mouse," by Jody, age 11.

---

Emotional Content 1: solitary subject portrayed as isolated, suicidal, and tearful
Self-Image 1: Connie may identify the bride with herself
Ability to Select 5: imaginative, well-organized idea, implies more than is visible
Ability to Combine 5: takes into account the entire drawing area
Ability to Represent 5: highly expressive and suggestive

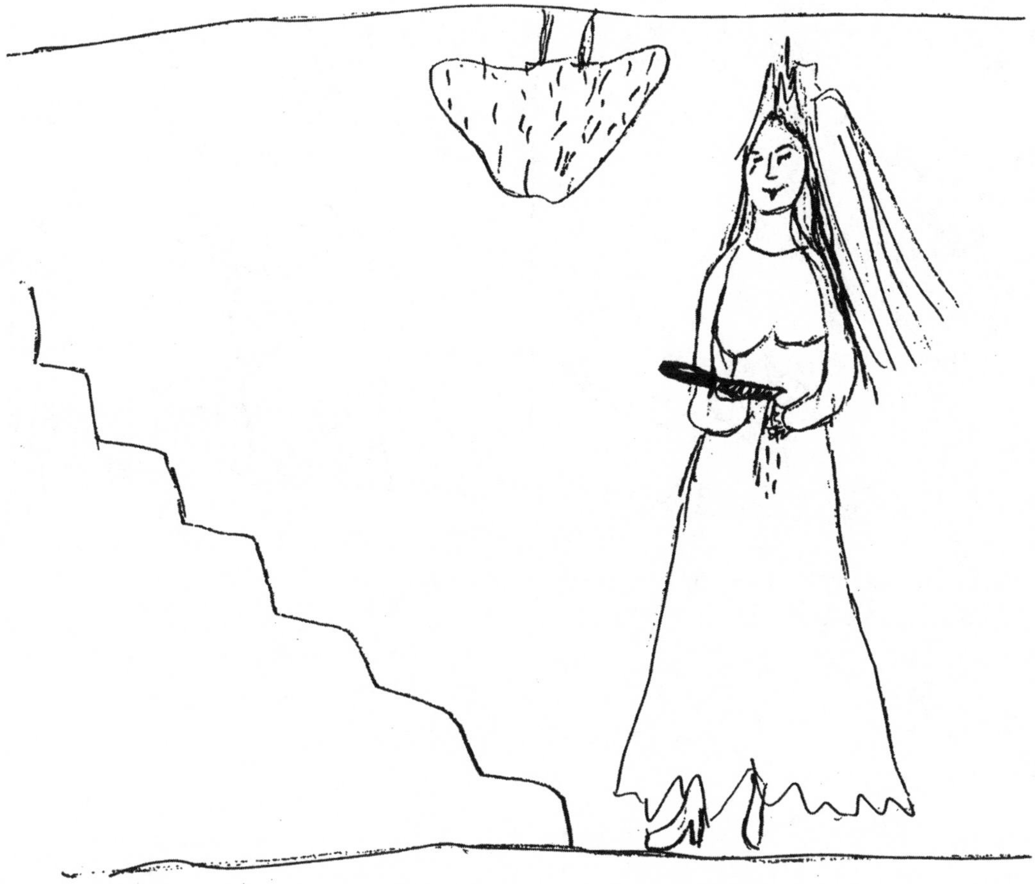

Figure 7.20.  "The Dying Bride," by Connie, age 14, no impairments.

Emotional Content 1: life-threatening relationships
Self-Image 3: unclear; John could identify himself with his predators, victims, or the narrator
Ability to Select 5: imaginative, well-organized idea, uses abstract words
Ability to Combine 5: two drawings, different subjects illustrate the title
Ability to Represent 5: original, expressive

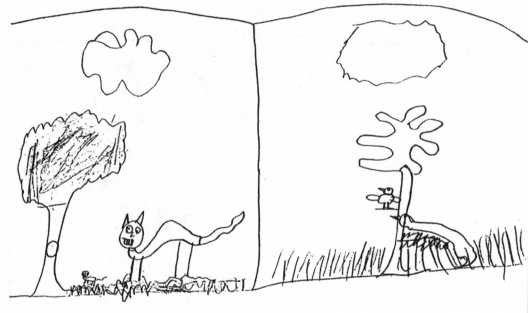

Figure 7.21. "Victims of Death," by John, age 8, no impairments.

Emotional Content 3: unemotional

Self-Image 3: unclear; Betty may identify with the girl

Ability to Select 2: girl and dog are related by the leash, and by placement

Ability to Combine 3: girl and dog are related along an implied baseline

Ability to Represent 3: girl and dog are restructured

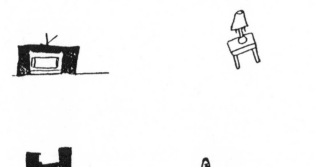

Figure 7.22.   Untitled Drawing by Betty, age 13, severe sensorineural and receptive language disabilities; hearing loss 78 dB in her better ear.

Emotional Content 3: both dog and cat are smiling

Self-Image 3: Caroline seems to be the invisible narrator

Ability to Select 3: functional

Ability to Combine 3: implies baseline

Ability to Represent 3: restructures stimulus drawings

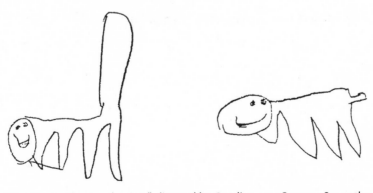

Figure 7.23.   "The Dog Is Chasing the Cat," dictated by Caroline, age 3 years, 9 months.

Emotional Content 1: lethal relationship

Self-Image 5: powerful, achieving goals

Use of Humor 1.5: lethal but not morbid

Ability to Select 5: conceptual level, imaginative, well-organized idea

Ability to Combine 5: a series of two or more drawings

Ability to Represent 5: transformational, highly original, expressive, playful, suggestive

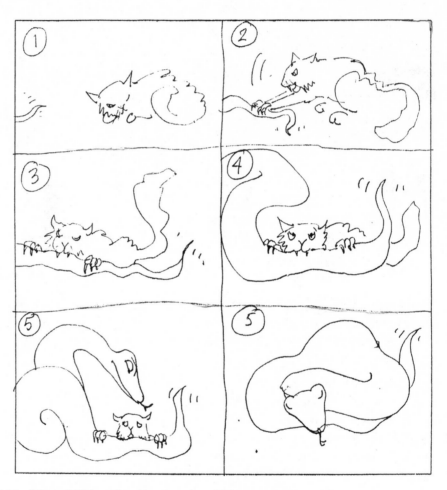

Figure 7.24. "Biting Off More Than You Can Chew," by a young man.

Emotional Content 3: moderately positive, solitary subject, fortunate but passive

Self-Image 3: absent

Use of Humor 2: disparaging

Ability to Select 3: descriptive rather than abstract

Ability to Combine 2: attempts to show relationship with dotted line

Ability to Represent 3: moderately original and expressive

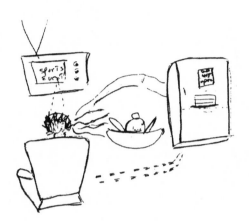

Figure 7.25. "Fat Couch Potato Watching Sports-Event . . . ," by an older woman.

Emotional Content 3.5: the snake is frustrated, the mouse escapes

Self-Image 5: Bruce seems to identify with the successful mouse

Use of Humor 4: resilient, mouse overcomes adversity

Ability to Select 5: imaginative, well-organized idea

Ability to Combine 3: beyond the baseline level

Ability to Represent 5: original, expressive, playful

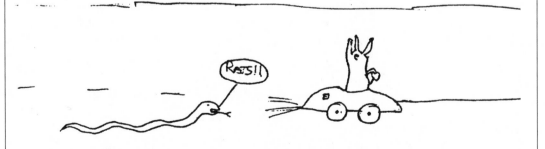

Figure 7.26. "The Great Escape," by Bruce, age 16, no impairments.

Emotional Content 2: stressful relationships
Self-Image 3: ambivalent with unclear outcome
Use of Humor 1.5: lethal but not morbid
Ability to Select 5: imaginative, well-organized idea
Ability to Combine 5: series of drawings
Ability to Represent 5: highly original,
     expressive, playful

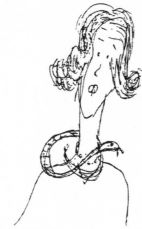

Figure 7.27. "Now They Can't Snatch My Gold Chain," by a young
woman.

Emotional Content 5
Self-Image 3: ambiguous
Use of Humor 5
Ability to Select 5
Ability to Combine 3
Ability to Represent 5

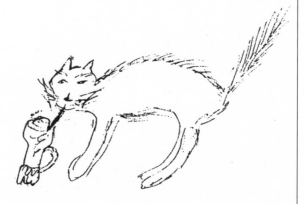

Figure 7.28. "Cat Sip or Cat-a-Tonic," by a young man.

Emotional Content 1
Self-Image 5
Use of Humor 1.5
Ability to Select 5
Ability to Combine 5
Ability to Represent 5

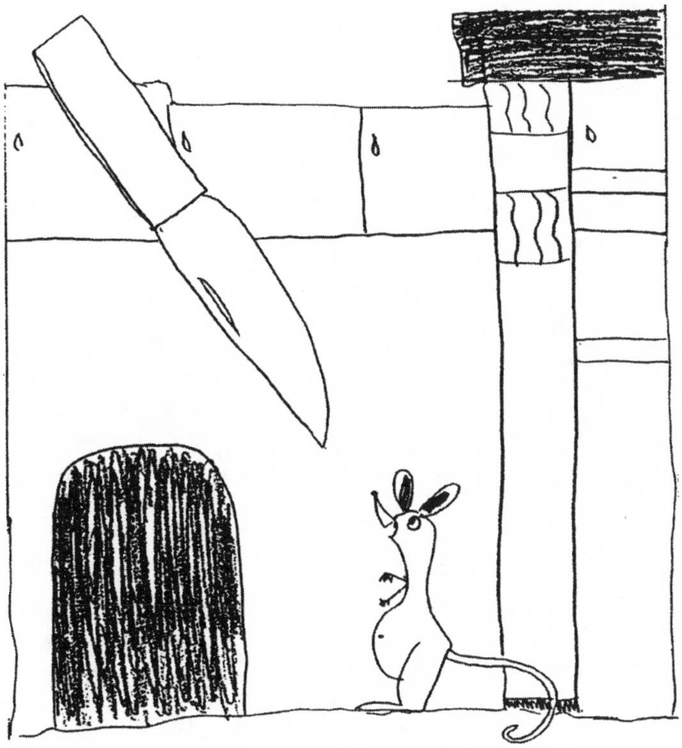

Figure 7.29. "The Great Mouse Murder," by Roy, age 17.

Emotional Content 2
Self-Image 2.5
Use of Humor 2.5
Ability to Select 5
Ability to Combine 4
Ability to Represent 5

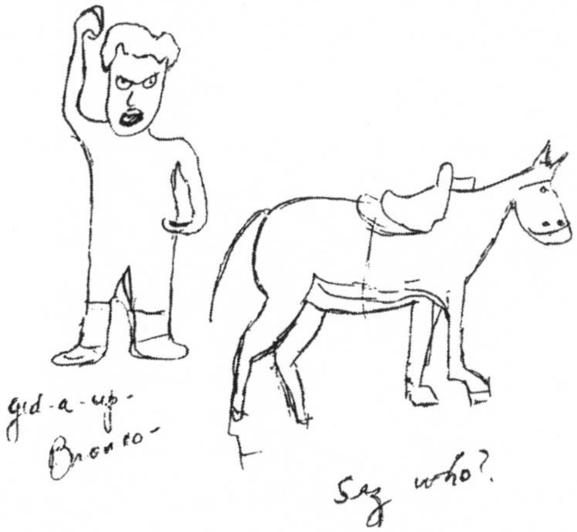

Figure 7.30. "Giddiap!" by a young man.

★ Note: Figures 7.30–7.36 were responses to the Form C stimulus drawings; see chapter 13.

Emotional Content 1
Self-Image 3
Use of Humor 1.5
Ability to Select 5
Ability to Combine 5
Ability to Represent 5

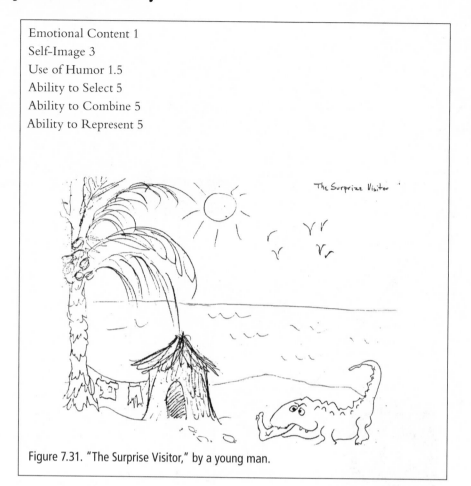

Figure 7.31. "The Surprise Visitor," by a young man.

Emotional Content 1
Self-Image 3
Use of Humor 1.5
Ability to Select 5
Ability to Combine 1
Ability to Represent 5

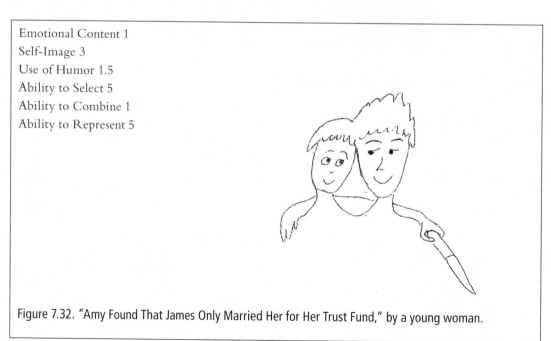

Figure 7.32. "Amy Found That James Only Married Her for Her Trust Fund," by a young woman.

Emotional Content 2
Self-Image 2
Use of Humor 2.5
Ability to Select 5
Ability to Combine 1
Ability to Represent 5

Figure 7.33.  "I Am a Pisces, So Where Is the Other Fish?" by a senior woman.

Emotional Content 3
Self-Image 3
Use of Humor 2.5
Ability to Select 5
Ability to Combine 3
Ability to Represent 5

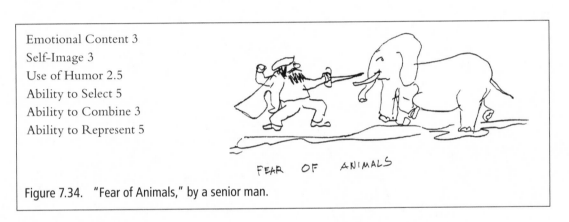

Figure 7.34.  "Fear of Animals," by a senior man.

Emotional Content 2
Self-Image 3.5
Use of Humor 4
Ability to Select 5
Ability to Combine 5
Ability to Represent 5

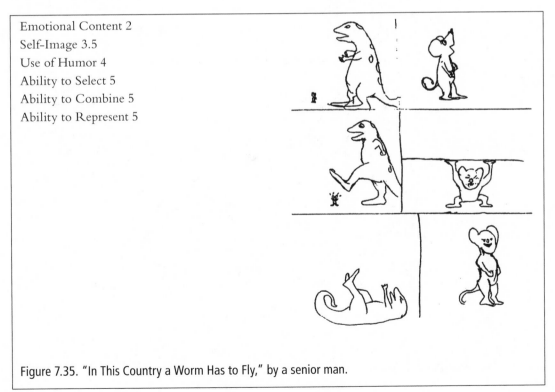

Figure 7.35. "In This Country a Worm Has to Fly," by a senior man.

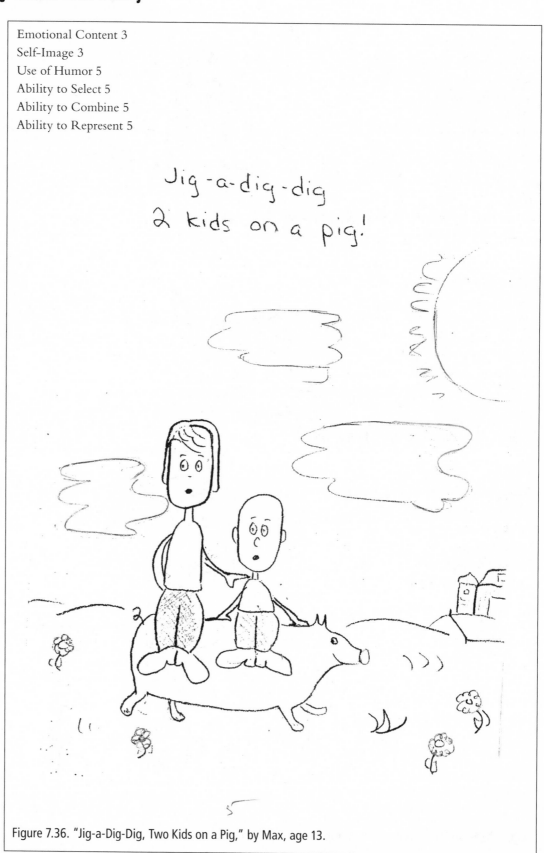

Emotional Content 3
Self-Image 3
Use of Humor 5
Ability to Select 5
Ability to Combine 5
Ability to Represent 5

Jig-a-dig-dig
2 kids on a pig!

Figure 7.36. "Jig-a-Dig-Dig, Two Kids on a Pig," by Max, age 13.

# Chapter 8

# The Reliability and Validity of the Silver Drawing Test

◇     ◇     ◇

In addition to reviewing previous studies of reliability and validity, this chapter reports new findings of interscorer reliability and significant correlations between standardized tests and the Drawing from Imagination task of the Silver Drawing Test (SDT).

To determine its reliability, the SDT has been administered to 1,425 children, adolescents, and adults by 22 art therapists, psychiatrists, psychologists, and classroom teachers. The respondents include 875 who had no known impairments, and 550 with brain injuries, emotional disturbances, learning disabilities, hearing and visual-motor disorders, as well as students performing below grade level residing in California, Florida, Idaho, Nebraska, New Jersey, New York, Pennsylvania, and Wisconsin, as well as in Canada and Russia.

## Interscorer Reliability

### 1. Comparing the Evaluations of Seven Judges

Seven studies of interscorer reliability have been conducted. In 1979, seven art therapists administered and scored responses to the SDT from children who were participating in the National Institute of Education Project discussed in chapter 6. Four of these were registered art therapists, and the other three had received master's degrees either in art therapy or education. After several training sessions, the judges scored the responses of six children who had been selected by school administrators for performing at least one year below grade level in reading or mathematics. Separate reliability coefficients were computed for each subtest.

*Results* The judges' ratings indicated a high degree of interscorer reliability. The coefficients were .93 in the Predictive Drawing task, .91 in the Drawing from Observation task, and .98 in the Drawing from Imagination task (see table 8.1).

## 2. Comparing the Evaluations of Six Judges

In a previous study, six judges scored the SDT responses of 11 children with visual-motor disabilities (Silver & Lavin, 1977).

*Results* An analysis of variance indicated that the six judges had a similar frame of reference and displayed a high degree of agreement in scoring the tests. The reliability coefficient was .852 in ability to select, combine, and represent (drawing from imagination), and .944 in spatial orientation (drawing from observation, sequencing, and conserving).

## 3. Comparing Evaluations of Self-Image and Emotional Content Scores by Five Judges

In a recent study, five judges evaluated responses to the Drawing from Imagination task in order to determine reliability for the self-image scale and the emotional content scale. Four judges were registered art therapists, and the fifth was a graduate student in a university art therapy program.

The judges scored five responses selected at random from a group of 15 responses by 7 males and 8 females (4 children, 5 adolescents, and 6 adults). The judges met for approximately one hour to practice scoring the 10 unselected responses, then independently scored the 5 selected responses. The ratings for each of the two scales were analyzed separately.

The judges used the intraclass correlation (ICC) statistic, a measure of interscorer reliability; the results obtained are shown in table 8.2.

| Table 8.1  Interscorer Reliability Coefficients for SDT Subtests by Seven Judges | |
|---|---|
| Predictive Drawing | .93 |
| Drawing from Observation | .91 |
| Drawing from Imagination | .98 |

| Table 8.2  Interscorer Reliability for the Self-Image and Emotional Content Scales for Five Judges | |
|---|---|
| Scale | ICC |
| Emotional Content Scale | 0.94 |
| Self-Image Scale | 0.74 |

These data show strong reliability for the emotional content scale and moderate reliability for the self-image scale. Thus, it appears that the scales show interscorer reliability.

The following studies were undertaken to determine the adequacy of the SDT scoring guidelines for judges who did not participate in training sessions.

## 4. Comparing Evaluations of Cognitive Skill by a Registered Art Therapist with No Special Training and the Author

The director of an art therapy program in Pennsylvania scored test booklets administered to 16 tenth-grade students and 20 fourth-grade students. He used the guidelines provided in a preliminary version of the SDT manual. The booklets were subsequently scored by the author (who had not met the director).

All correlations were found significant, five at the .01 level and one at the .05 level, as shown in table 8.3. These data show moderate reliability. They suggest that the scoring guidelines alone are adequate when used by a registered art therapist, and that training sessions for such examiners are unnecessary.

## 5. Comparing Evaluations of Cognitive Skill by Another Registered Therapist with No Special Training and the Author

A registered art therapist in Virginia who learned to score the SDT by reading its manual administered the SDT to nine hospitalized adults with mental disabilities. The art therapist and the author scored the test booklets.

The judges displayed a high degree of agreement in scoring the tests, as shown in table 8.4. These data show strong reliability, again suggesting that training sessions for registered art therapists are not necessary.

Table 8.3 Correlations for Subtests Scored by a Registered Art Therapist with No Special Training and the Author

| Subtest | r | p |
|---|---|---|
| Tenth-Graders (n = 16) | | |
| Predictive Drawing | .71 | .01 |
| Drawing from Observation | .81 | .01 |
| Drawing from Imagination | .79 | .01 |
| Fourth-Graders (n = 20) | | |
| Predictive Drawing | .86 | .01 |
| Drawing from Observation | .45 | .05 |
| Drawing from Imagination | .65 | .01 |

Table 8.4 Correlations for Subtests Scored by an Art Therapist with No Special Training and the Author (n = 9)

| Subtest | r | p |
|---|---|---|
| Predictive Drawing | .99 | .01 |
| Drawing from Observation | .89 | .01 |
| Drawing from Imagination | .91 | .01 |
| Total | .96 | .01 |

| Table 8.5 Interscorer Reliability Coefficients of Evaluations by Five Judges |
| --- |
| Mean = 32.55 |
| SD = 4.5 |
| $r$ = .66 |
| $p < .01$ |

### 6. Comparing Evaluations by a Classroom Teacher, a Psychotherapist, and Three Art Therapists

In revising the SDT manual for the second edition, changes were made in the wording of the scoring guidelines in an attempt to make scoring more precise. To determine whether the changes would affect interscorer reliability, 5 judges used the revised guidelines to score the performances of 10 third-graders in a public school in Nebraska. The judges included the children's teacher in Nebraska, who learned to score the SDT by reading its manual; a psychotherapist in Florida; and three art therapists in Pennsylvania. Scorers A and B were registered art therapists who had learned about the SDT by reading its manual, and scorer C was a graduate student who learned about the test from scorer A. None of the scorers had met the author.

Reliability coefficients were computed for their evaluations of the total test scores. Significant correlations at the .01 level were found, as indicated in table 8.5, suggesting that training sessions also are unnecessary for teachers and psychotherapists.

### 7. Interscorer Reliability of the Scale for Assessing the Use of Humor

As reported in chapter 3, a scorer reliability coefficient of 0.86 was found for the Draw a Story (DAS) humor scale. Since it is the same scale used for assessing humorous responses to the SDT Drawing from Imagination task, the scale appears to be reliable.

## Retest Reliability

To determine the test/retest reliability of the SDT, it was administered on two occasions to groups of children and adolescents. Their responses were scored and reliability coefficients computed.

### 8. Comparing Performance Scores of 12 Adolescents with Learning Disabilities after Approximately One Month

Moser (1980) used the SDT in her doctoral project, administering it twice to 12 adolescents with learning disabilities with a time lapse of approximately one month, and computing reliability coefficients for each subtest. All correlations were significant at the .05 level. The test/retest reliability scores are strong in the Drawing from Observation task and the "ability to represent spatial concepts" (Moser's term for the Predictive Drawing task), but weak in the Drawing from Imagination task, as shown in table 8.6.

Table 8.6 Test–Retest Reliability Coefficients of Adolescents with Learning Disabilities (Moser, 1980)

| Subtest | r | p |
|---|---|---|
| Predictive Drawing | .8036 | .05 |
| Drawing from Observation | .8401 | .05 |
| Drawing from Imagination | .5637 | .05 |

## 9. Comparing the Performance Scores of 10 Children after Approximately One Month

A teacher in an urban public school in Nebraska administered the SDT to all children in a third-grade class in November 1989. She administered the test again in December 1989 to 10 of the children, whom she described as the "top students across the board." Limiting the retest group to top scorers limits the reliability of the findings.

Five judges scored the responses. To ensure that the judges would score blindly, the students' drawings were identified only by first names: the first test performance by each examinee was identified by the child's real name; the second, by a fictitious name beginning with the same letter of the alphabet. For example, Sandra's second booklet was named Susie; Andrew's second booklet, Arthur. Thus, the judges assumed they were scoring one test performance by each of 20 children but were actually scoring two test performances by each of 10 children.

Moderate correlations were found in the Drawing from Imagination task and in total test scores. Low correlations were found in the Drawing from Observation task. No significant correlations were found in the Predictive Drawing task, as shown in table 8.7.

The inconsistencies in test/retest correlations suggest that the Drawing from Imagination task may be an unstable construct for adolescents but not children with learning disabilities, whereas the Predictive Drawing task may be unstable for children but not for adolescents.

A review of the children's responses to the Predictive Drawing task found that in the retest, two children failed to draw any lines in the tilted bottle, thus lowering their scores from 4 points in the first test to 0 in the retest. Two other children apparently had learned that water remains horizontal regardless of the tilt of its container, raising their scores from 1 point on the first test to 5 points on the second test.

Table 8.7 Test–Retest Reliability Coefficients of Third-Graders

| Subtest | r | p |
|---|---|---|
| Predictive Drawing | .08 | ns |
| Drawing from Observation | .61 | .05 |
| Drawing from Imagination | .70 | .02 |
| Total | .72 | .02 |

In addition, one child scored 5 points in the first test, drawing a sequence of descending lines in the soda glasses without corrections. In the retest, however, she erased the lines she drew in the glasses, thus lowering her score to 3 points.

Scores in the Predictive Drawing task are based on observations by Piaget and Inhelder (1967), who have found that children use trial and error when they do not know the solutions to problems; when they do know the solutions, however, they proceed systematically without resorting to trial and error. As this child had represented a sequence systematically in the first test, it seems unlikely that her erasures in the second test reflected trial and error. It may be, instead, that the erasures reflected feelings of insecurity or a desire for perfection. At any event, the variations in retest scores suggest that the visual-spatial abilities measured by the Predictive Drawing task may be unstable in this age group. This test/retest reliability underestimates the reliability of the test.

# Correlations between the Silver Drawing Test and Traditional Tests of Creativity and Achievement

## 10. Correlations among the Silver Drawing Test, the Torrance Test of Creative Thinking, and the Creativity Assessment Packet

Two Russian psychiatrists, Kopytin and Svistovskaya, found significant correlations between the SDT and the Torrance Test of Creative Thinking (Torrance, 1984) as well as The Creativity Assessment Packet (Williams, 1980). These investigators tested children and adolescents in Russia, where the SDT had been translated, standardized, and published in 2001.

They calculated correlations between the students' scores in the ability to represent, one of the three scales in the SDT Drawing from Imagination task, as well as their scores on the creativity tests. The scale for assessing ability to represent was based on the premise that examinees whose responses to the Drawing from Imagination task show originality, expressiveness, and playfulness, and have high levels of creative ability, score 5 points; and that lower levels, such as restructuring or imitating stimulus drawings or stereotypes, can be inferred and scored. In addition, these investigators calculated correlations between the students' total SDT scores and total scores on the two creativity tests.

The Creativity Assessment Packet (CAP) was chosen because it assesses creativity as a complex characteristic comprising both cognitive and personality factors, and includes three parts. The first is the Test of Divergent Thinking, in which respondents are asked to complete 12 stimulus drawings. This test is designed to assess the cognitive factors of creativity. In the second part, the Test of Creative Characteristics of Personality, respondents answer 50 questions designed to evaluate personality features associated with creativity. In the third part, teachers and parents are asked to give their opinions about the children's creative potential.

The subjects of the study included 26 children and adolescents, ages 9 to 16 (15 boys and 11 girls), in a residential school in Russia. The authors of this report served as judges. Both were initially trained as psychiatrists, and later took training in art therapy. After the responses were scored, they were examined for creativity.

*Results*    Stronger correlations emerged between the creativity tests and the ability to represent than total test scores of the SDT, supporting the premise that the ability to represent scale can serve to identify creative ability. Correlations between ability to represent in the SDT Drawing from Imagination task and most of the creativity tests were significant either at the .05 or the .01 levels. The most significant correlation (.01) appeared between ability to represent and the CAP's Test of Divergent Thinking. The only nonsignificant correlation was found between ability to represent and the CAP's Creative Characteristics of Personality test, as shown in table 8.8.

In total test scores, correlations between SDT total scores and scores on the CAP Test of Divergent Thinking were found significant at the .01 level.

No significant correlations were found between SDT scores and scores on the CAP's Creative Characteristics of Personality test and its Scale for Parents. Moderately significant correlations at the .05 level were found between total SDT scores and scores on the Torrance Test of Creative Thinking and the CAP Scale for Teachers, as shown in table 8.9.

Kopytin and Svistovskaya have concluded that the SDT, especially in the ability to represent, is more sensitive to cognitive factors of creativity than personality factors.

**Table 8.8  Correlations between Scores on the SDT Drawing from Imagination Task (Ability to Represent) and Traditional Tests of Creativity**

| Test | Mean | SD | r | p |
|---|---|---|---|---|
| CAP Test of Divergent Thinking | 73.7 | 9.5 | 0.60 | 0.01 |
| CAP Creative Characteristics of Personality Test | 64.3 | 11.0 | 0.18 | n.s. |
| CAP Scale for Teachers | 40.1 | 14.4 | 0.34 | 0.05 |
| CAP Scale for Parents | 49.9 | 10.4 | 0.39 | 0.05 |
| Torrance Test of Creative Thinking | 53.7 | 20.7 | 0.38 | 0.05 |
| Silver Drawing Test, Drawing from Imagination Task (Ability to Represent) | 2.7 | 1.0 | | |

| Table 8.9 Correlations between the SDT (Total Scores) and Traditional Tests of Creativity | | | | |
|---|---|---|---|---|
| | CAP Test of Divergent Thinking | CAP Creative Characteristics of Personality Test | CAP Scale for Teachers | CAP Scale for Parents | Torrance Test of Creative Thinking |
| SDT Total Scores | 0.51 | 0.04 | 0.35 | 0.29 | 0.35 |

### 11. Hayes's Finding of Correlations between the Silver Drawing Test and the Science Research Associates Reading Test

Karen Hayes (1978), a classroom teacher in an urban parochial school, had been troubled that the amount of time given to art education had been diminishing each year and even eliminated altogether by budget cutting or "back-to-basics zealots." She believed it was important for primary teachers and art teachers to become aware of similarities between the mental processes involved in drawing and reading and decided to devote her master's thesis to examining relationships between children's drawings and reading scores.

*Procedures*   Hayes administered the SDT to 75 children in grades 1 to 3, and then compared their SDT scores with their reading scores. She correlated the SDT scores of first graders with their scores on the Science Research Associates (SRA) Informal Reading Inventory and the scores of second- and third-graders with their scores on the SRA Reading Achievement Test, Form F, Primary II. Homeroom teachers selected at random 25 children from each of the three grades to participate in the study. The children were then grouped as high, middle, or low reading achievers, as determined by the SRA Informal Reading Inventory and the SRA Achievement Series Test. The children had not been exposed to any formal art classes, due to a reduced budget, and if they received any art experience previously, it was provided by classroom teachers.

The children lived in predominantly middle-class homes in the Bronx, New York, and spoke English at home. They ranged in age from 6 to 9 years; 38 were girls, 37 were boys.

Hayes administered the SDT to approximately 10 children at a time, over a period of two weeks, administering it individually to students who had been absent from their groups. Her study attempted to answer the following questions:

Is there a correlation between children's ability to associate and represent concepts as found in their ability to read and ability to draw from imagination?

Do reading scores correlate with ability to perceive and represent spatial relationships when drawing from observation?

Do reading scores correlate with ability to order sequentially and to represent
spatial concepts through predictive drawing?

Is the relationship between performances, as measured by reading scores and scores
on the SDT Drawing from Imagination task, stronger for boys than for girls?

Hayes used the Spearman rank-order formula to determine the strength of correlations, and compared correlation coefficients for boys and girls to determine whether
gender differences emerged.

*Results* In all three grades, significant correlations emerged between reading
achievement scores and Drawing from Imagination task scores. Since all correlation
coefficients were statistically significant, the null hypothesis was rejected at the .05
level of significance ($r$ = .945, .657, and .668 for grades 1 to 3, respectively). The
relationship between reading ability and the SDT was stronger for girls than boys in
grades 2 and 3. On the other hand, correlations between the Drawing from Observation task and reading scores were significant for third-graders only, indicating that
Drawing from Observation scores did not correlate consistently with reading scores.
The finding of one strong correlation suggested that further investigation would be
useful.

The correlations between the Predictive Drawing task and reading achievement
also were inconsistent, with weak correlation for the first grade and no significance
for the second and third grades. The relationship between reading and artistic performance, as measured by Drawing from Imagination, was stronger for boys in the first
grade, stronger for girls than for boys in the second and third grades.

*Concluding Observations* Hayes noted that the Drawing from Imagination task provided insight into the child's personality and concepts of reality, in addition to the
correlations found between ability to read and represent concepts. She concluded that
art instruction should be an integral part of the primary school curriculum, since the
cognitive skills needed in art do correlate with the cognitive skills needed in reading
and other academic subjects. She suggested that some other testing device be used to
assess reading ability rather than the SRA Achievement Series.

## 12. Anderson's Finding of Correlations between the SDT and the Gates-MacGinitie Reading Comprehension Test

Victoria Anderson (2001) examined relationships between the cognitive skills used
in comprehending prose and in composing a drawing from imagination. She hypothesized that positive correlations would be found between scores on the SDT Drawing
from Imagination task and scores on the Gates-MacGinitie Reading Test. This standardized reading test is used annually in an urban, public, magnet middle school in

Pennsylvania to measure the reading comprehension of its students. The test assesses ability to read paragraphs of prose, and ability to answer multiple-choice questions.

The language arts teacher administered both tests (in varying order) to approximately 250 students in each grade during the same class period. Twenty-four of these students volunteered to have their scores correlated in order to explore relationships between reading comprehension and drawing from imagination.

The students, ages 11 to 13, included 14 sixth-graders, 4 seventh-graders, and 6 eighth-graders. Of the 50-minute period, 35 minutes were devoted to the reading test, and 15 minutes to the SDT. Reading test scores were based on grade-equivalent norms. Scores on both tests were correlated using Pearson's $r$.

The correlation for the 24 students yielded results that were significant at the .01 level of probability ($r = .53$, $p < .01$), showing with 99% certainty that a significant relationship exists between scores on both measures.

Anderson's study seems to support the validity of using the SDT to assess the cognitive skills considered fundamental in comprehending written language, and provides interesting observations for future investigation.

### 13. Swanson's Finding of Correlations between the Silver Drawing Test and the Science Research Associates Survey of Basic Skills Ability

Joan Swanson, a school teacher in Nebraska, volunteered to administer the SDT to 15 of her students (Silver, 1990). The students, ages 13 and 14, comprised one-half of her eighth grade class in a rural public school. Since the class previously had been divided for periods of music and art, she administered the SDT to students attending the art period, and then sent the test booklets to me for scoring. In addition, she sent, in a sealed envelope, the students' scores on the SRA Survey of Basic Skills Ability, administered the previous spring to assess ability and progress. I gave the sealed envelope and the SDT scores to a statistician who analyzed the results.

*Results*    The statistician found significant correlations between the SRA scores and total SDT scores, as well as two of the three SDT tasks, Predictive Drawing and Drawing from Imagination, as shown in table 8.10. She did not find significant correlations between the SRA and the SDT Drawing from Observation task.

| Table 8.10  Correlations between Scores on the SDT and the SRA Survey of Basic Skills Ability | | | | |
|---|---|---|---|---|
| Subtest | Mean | SD | $r$ | $p$ |
| Predictive Drawing | 11.4 | 1.8 | 0.52 | 0.05 |
| Drawing from Observation | 12.2 | 2.4 | 0.51 | n.s. |
| Drawing from Imagination | 9.8 | 2.5 | 0.68 | 0.01 |
| Total | 33.4 | 5.0 | 0.76 | 0.01 |
| SRA Survey of Basic Skills Ability | 104.7 | 9.8 | | |

## 14. Comparing SDT Scores with Scores on the Metropolitan Achievement Test (Reading and Mathematics)

Madeline Altabe, PhD, used correlational analysis to determine whether the SDT was related to school achievement, as measured by the Metropolitan Achievement Test (MAT). She compared the three SDT cognitive subtest scores of 40 children with their reading and mathematics scores on the MAT, which had been administered previously by school personnel. The children attended grades 1 to 3 in a suburban public school in a low- to middle-income neighborhood in New York.

*Results*    The SDT and MAT scales appear to be related, even though the MAT is a language-oriented test of scholastic achievement. The children's scores in the SDT Predictive Drawing, Drawing from Observation, and Drawing from Imagination tasks correlated significantly with their MAT reading and mathematics scores at the $p < .05$, $p < .01$, and $p < .001$ levels of significance, as shown in table 8.11.

Surprisingly, scores on the SDT Self-Image Scale also were related significantly to the MAT scores.

Table 8.11   Relationships between SDT Scales and MAT Scales among Elementary School Children in Grades 1 to 3 ($n = 40$)

| SDT Scales | MAT Reading | MAT Mathematics |
|---|---|---|
| Predictive Drawing | .39* | .42** |
| Drawing from Observation | .50*** | .44** |
| Drawing from Imagination | .36* | .34* |
| Emotional Content | n.s. | n.s. |
| Self-Image | .42** | .40** |

Notes: *$p < .05$; **$p < .01$, ***$p < .001$.

## 15. Horovitz-Darby's Findings of Concurrence with the Diagnostic Art Therapy Assessment

Ellen Horovitz-Darby, ART-BC, examined the role of clinical art therapy with deaf children and their families. She based her therapy on four assessments, including the SDT and the Diagnostic Art Therapy Assessment (DATA) (Horovitz-Darby, 1996). She reported a case study of a 10-year-old boy, which found concurrence between these assessments, yielding quantified information.

## 16. Correlations between Scores on the SDT and Scores on Six Traditional Tests of Intelligence and Achievement

In the National Institute of Education Project (Silver et al., 1980), we also compared SDT scores with scores on six traditional tests: the Canadian Cognitive Abilities Test (CCAT), the Otis-Lennon School Ability Test (OLSAT), the Wechsler Intelligence Scale for Children (WISC) Performance IQ, the Metropolitan Achievement

Test (MAT), the SRA Math Achievement Test, and the Iowa Test of Basic Skills (Composite).

Although significant relationships were found, the reliability coefficients with the Drawing from Imagination task were modest, and the correlations with the Drawing from Observation task were significant with only one traditional test, the Iowa Composite and Math Test, as shown in table 8.12.

The traditional tests are heavily weighted with verbal items not on the SDT. On the other hand, the SDT taps cognitive skills that they do not include. All the instruments assess intellectual ability, but use different techniques and emphasize language and visual-spatial cognitive skills to different extents.

What cannot be explained by correlations with these traditional tests may be explained by other cognitive strengths not measured by these tests. In the Predictive Drawing task, only 18 of 136 children received the highest possible scores, and 8 of the 18 had IQ scores ranging between 50 on the Stanford-Binet IQ Test and 140 on the Goodenough-Harris Draw-a-Man Test. Their ages ranged from 10 to 13.

The SDT has also been presented to audiences of teachers and other professionals. Surprisingly, some confused spatial relationships in the Drawing from Observation task, or drew houses perpendicular to the slope and even lines parallel to the sides of the tilted bottle in the Predictive Drawing task.

How can such failures be explained? It can't be lack of talent, because the drawing tasks call for more than art skills. Perhaps adults who say they can't draw a straight line have difficulty in processing spatial information, subtle cognitive dysfunctions that are easily overlooked because schools tend to emphasize verbal skills and it does not matter if students cannot draw. By the same token, subtle cognitive strengths may also be escaping detection. It may well be important to identify and evaluate these strengths

Table 8.12  Relationships among Scores on the SDT and Scores on the CCAT, the Otis-Lennon, the WISC Performance IQ, the MAT Reading, the SRA Math Achievement Test, and the Iowa Composite and Math Test

|  |  | Predictive Drawing |  | Drawing from Observation |  | Drawing from Imagination |  |
| --- | --- | --- | --- | --- | --- | --- | --- |
|  | n | r | p | r | p | r | p |
| CCAT | 25 | .33 | ns | .05 | ns | .50 | .01 |
| Otis-Lennon | 99 | .30 | .01 | .05 | ns | .39 | .01 |
| WISC Performance IQ | 65 | .33 | .01 | .16 | ns | .37 | .01 |
| MAT Reading | 76 | .32 | .01 | .03 | ns | .31 | .01 |
| SRA Math Achievement Test | 65 | .36 | .01 | −.15 | ns | .37 | .01 |
| Iowa Composite and Math Test | 20 | .11 | ns | .55 | .01 | .44 | .05 |

(and weaknesses) if they can be used in helping students with language deficits acquire concepts usually acquired verbally.

The results lend support to the hypothesis that the SDT measures cognitive skills through drawings rather than language. The Predictive Drawing task is based on the theory that it measures ability to predict and represent concepts of sequential order, horizontality, and verticality. The Drawing from Observation task is based on the theory that it measures ability to represent spatial relationships in height, width, and depth. The Drawing from Imagination task is based on the theory that it measures levels of ability to select, combine, and represent through images instead of words. These cognitive abilities seem relatively independent of language impairment and verbal-analytical thinking and, to some extent, independent of age.

The findings support the premise that the SDT can be used to identify cognitive skills in children with known language deficiencies—such as those with deafness, language impairment, learning disabilities, and other disadvantages—as well as adults who cannot communicate well verbally. These results also explain why we have found unexpected cognitive strengths in some children when using the SDT—strengths that do not appear on other tests.

## 17. Moser's Finding of Correlations among the Scores of 70 Adolescents with and without Learning Disabilities on the Silver Drawing Test and the Bender Visual Motor Gestalt, the Goodenough-Harris Draw-a-Man Test, and the Wechsler Adult Intelligence Scales Verbal and Performance IQ Tests

Joy Moser (1980) administered the SDT to 70 adolescents with and without learning disabilities, and compared their mean scores, as part of her doctoral project. The group with learning disabilities received lower scores than the control group to a degree significant at the .001 level of probability on the SDT and on the Goodenough-Harris Draw-a-Man Test at the .05 level, as shown in table 8.14.

These findings indicate that adolescents with and without learning disabilities who would be expected to differ in cognition do differ on the SDT.

Moser also compared the SDT scores of her subjects with learning disabilities with their scores on four other tests. She found significant correlations among the SDT total and subtest scores and scores on the Wechsler Adult Intelligence Scales (WAIS) Performance IQ test and the Goodenough-Harris Draw-a-Man Test at the .01 and .001 levels. Negative correlations were found among the SDT, the Bender Visual Motor Gestalt (BVMG), and the WAIS Verbal scores, as shown in tables 8.13 and 8.14.

The lack of correlations with the WAIS Verbal IQ supports the theory that the SDT does not measure verbal ability. Similarly, the lack of correlation with the

Table 8.13 Correlations among Scores on the SDT and Draw-a-Man Tests by 36 Adolescents with Learning Disabilities and 34 Control Group Adolescents

| Variable | Experimental Mean (n = 36) | SD | Control Mean (n = 34) | SD | t | p |
|---|---|---|---|---|---|---|
| Predictive Drawing | 3.28 | 1.02 | 4.65 | .63 | −6.98 | .001 |
| Drawing from Observation | 3.93 | 1.20 | 4.9 | .30 | −4.84 | .001 |
| Drawing from Imagination | 2.48 | 1.30 | 3.63 | 1.14 | −4.01 | .001 |
| Total | 3.20 | .95 | 4.39 | .54 | −6.65 | .001 |
| Draw-a-Man | 40.26 | 10.59 | 46.95 | 9.50 | −2.45 | .05 |

Table 8.14 Correlation Matrix between Scores on the SDT and the Draw-a-Man, BVMG, and WAIS Performance Tests by 36 Learning-Disabled Adolescents

| Variable | 1 | 2 | 3 | 4 | 5 | 6 | 7 | 8 |
|---|---|---|---|---|---|---|---|---|
| 1 Drawing from Imagination | 1.00 | | | | | | | |
| 2 Drawing from Observation | .45** | 1.00 | | | | | | |
| 3 Predictive Drawing | .62*** | .22 | 1.00 | | | | | |
| 4 Silver Test Total | .88*** | .71*** | .75*** | 1.00 | | | | |
| 5 Draw-a-Man | .75*** | .31* | .62*** | .72*** | 1.00 | | | |
| 6 BMVG | −.59*** | −.17 | −.42 | −.50*** | −.37** | 1.00 | | |
| 7 WAIS Verbal | −.04 | .18 | −.01 | .02 | −.12 | −.01 | 1.00 | |
| 8 WAIS Performance | .59*** | .37** | .50*** | .60*** | .60*** | −.45** | .01 | 1.00 |

Notes: *$p = .05$; **$p = .01$; ***$p = .001$

BMVG supports the theory that the SDT measures conceptual skills and creativity. The BVMG asks examinees to copy nine abstract designs and, as stated in its name, is a measure of visual–motor skills, whereas the SDT gives copying its lowest score and originality its highest.

In presenting the WAIS Verbal Scale, the examiner reads questions aloud and examinees respond orally, thus requiring auditory–verbal input and verbal output. In presenting the SDT, the examiner can bypass language with pantomime, and examinees receive and respond to directions nonverbally through images. Although the Drawing from Imagination task also asks for verbal responses, it can be scored without them.

Conversely, positive correlations between the SDT, the Draw–a–Man, and the WAIS Performance Scale suggest that these measures tap similar abilities and assess similar constructs. As no correlations were found between the SDT and the BVMG and the SDT and the WAIS Verbal, they seem to assess different constructs.

## Concluding Remarks

This chapter has reviewed 17 studies that found interscorer reliability, retest reliability, or significant correlations between the SDT and traditional, language-oriented tests of intelligence or achievement.

Chapter 9 reviews the normative data that were developed.

# Chapter 9

# Normative Data

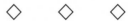

**N**orms make it possible to compare individual scores with typical scores. This chapter presents normative data so that responses to the Silver Drawing Test (SDT) by particular individuals can be compared with others. For rough estimates, individual scores above the mean indicate above-average performance; scores below the mean indicate below-average performance. For more precise information, percentile ranks and $t$ scores are provided in tables 9.8 to 9.10.

The norms are based on responses by 812 presumably normal children, adolescents, young adults, and senior adults. More than 700 people with various disabilities also responded to the drawing tasks; their scores are not included in the normative data but are presented in other chapters, as are the scores of respondents outside the United States.

To help develop these norms, art therapists and educators volunteered to administer the SDT to children, adolescents, young adults, and seniors who resided in California, Connecticut, Florida, Missouri, Nebraska, New Hampshire, New Jersey, New Mexico, New York, Pennsylvania, Texas, and Wisconsin as well as in Canada. The children and adolescents attended heterogeneous classes in 13 public elementary and secondary schools and one private elementary and high school. They included urban schools in Nebraska and New York, suburban schools in New York and Pennsylvania, and rural schools in Nebraska and Ontario. The schools were in low-, middle-, and high-income neighborhoods. The students came from various ethnic backgrounds and were of Caucasian, African American, and Hispanic descent. This information is not recorded in the normative data.

The 241 adults who responded to the drawing tasks in the United States included undergraduate and graduate students, art therapists, teachers, social workers, and retirees. The younger adults, ages 20 to 50 (average age, 28.7 years) responded to the SDT while participating in workshops or college audiences in Nebraska, New York, and Wisconsin. The senior adults lived independently in their own homes or retirement communities and had volunteered to respond to the tasks while participating in recreational or other programs in Florida and New York. Although the seniors had been asked only to provide their ages in 5-year increments beginning at age 65, 20 of them gave their actual ages, which averaged 80.8 years.

## Scores for Assessing Emotions and Cognitive Skills

The SDT scores and percentile ranks showed gradual improvement with age. Where reversals occurred in the prevailing upward trend, they were small and well within chance limits for these sample sizes.

The younger adults had higher cognitive scores than the high school students in each subtest. They also had higher scores than the senior adults in the Predictive Drawing task but lower scores in the Drawing from Imagination task.

In addition to mean scores, we examined responses to the SDT for the frequency of each of the scores. Subjects included 163 male and 189 female children, adolescents, and adults.

SDT responses by small samples of gifted children also were examined. They included all children previously identified as gifted in one fourth-grade class and one combined fifth- and sixth-grade class. Although each scored above the norm in each task, and their mean scores exceeded the mean scores of their classmates, the number of children previously identified as gifted was too small to quantify for statistical analysis. This preliminary exploration suggests that a study of larger numbers of gifted children would be worthwhile.

## Emotional Content, Self-Image, and the Use of Humor

In most age groups, males tended to have lower, more negative scores than females in emotional content than self-image, as well as more negative themes and fantasies. Conversely, the sample of men had higher, more positive self-image scores than the sample of women, but high school girls had slightly higher self-image scores than did high school boys. Girls in grades 1 to 8 had higher mean scores than boys in emotional content; boys had higher mean scores in self-image. The neutral, 3-point score predominated across genders in both emotional content and self-image.

In emotional content, more than three times as many males scored 1 point—17% of the males compared with 5% of the females—portraying life-threatening relationships, or sad/helpless solitary subjects. On the other hand, more females scored 4 and 5 points, indicating that 27% of the females compared with 15% of the males portrayed friendly relationships or fortunate/passive subjects, and 13% of the females compared with 9% of the males portrayed caring relationships or effective/powerful subjects.

In self-image scores, the converse emerged. Although the neutral, 3-point score predominated, more males than females scored 4 and 5 points: 18% of the males compared with 12% of the females seemed to identify with subjects portrayed as powerful, loved, assaultive, destructive, or achieving goals; 18% of the males compared with 13% of the females seemed to identify with subjects portrayed as fortunate but passive.

In the use of humor, 16% of the 888 responses to the Drawing from Imagination task suggested humorous intent. The humor was predominantly negative; 69% responded with negative humor (lethal, morbid, or disparaging) compared with only 22% positive (resilient or playful) responses. In addition, negative humor appeared significantly more often in male than female responses, as discussed in chapters 3 and 14.

## Mean Scores and Gender Frequencies

Table 9.1 presents mean cognitive scores based on age and grade levels; tables 9.2 and 9.3 present the mean scores in emotional content and self-image. Tables 9.4 and 9.5 present frequencies of female and male scores in emotional content; tables 9.6 and 9.7 present gender frequencies in self-image. Tables 9.8 through 9.11 show percentile ranks and $t$ score conversions for the Predictive Drawing, Drawing from Observation, and Drawing from Imagination tasks, and for total SDT scores.

| | | | Table 9.1 Mean Scores (and Standard Deviations) for SDT Cognitive Skills | | | |
|---|---|---|---|---|---|---|
| Grade | Age | $n$ | Mean Score, Predictive Drawing | Mean Score, Drawing from Observation | Mean Score, Drawing from Imagination | Mean Score Totals |
| 1 | 6–7 | 22 | 4.82 | 6.27 | 7.55 | 18.91 |
| 2 | 7–8 | 82 | 7.92 | 8.05 | 8.41 | 24.38 |
| 3 | 8–9 | 127 | 8.51 | 9.02 | 8.78 | 26.81 |
| 4 | 9–10 | 106 | 8.54 | 8.36 | 10.01 | 26.91 |
| 5 | 10–11 | 66 | 9.32 | 9.42 | 9.24 | 27.98 |
| 6 | 11–12 | 27 | 8.87 | 10.27 | 10.08 | 29.22 |
| 7 | 12–13 | 26 | 9.88 | 10.04 | 11.47 | 31.39 |
| 8 | 13–14 | 39 | 11.74 | 12.32 | 11.01 | 35.07 |
| High School | | 76 | 10.93 (2.82) | 10.22 (3.68) | 10.89 (2.28) | |
| Young Adult | | 162 | 12.50 (2.19) | 13.88 (1.61) | 12.64 (2.11) | |
| Senior | | 79 | 11.31 (2.90) | n/a | 14.34 (0.83) | |

# The Silver Drawing Test and Draw a Story

Table 9.2   Mean Scores (and Standard Deviations) for SDT Emotional Content and Self-Image Scales in Responses by Children in Elementary School Grades 1 to 8 (112 Boys, 96 Girls)

| Grade | Ages | Emotional Content | Self-Image |
|---|---|---|---|
| First Grade | 6–7 | | |
| Boys (8) | | 1.63 (0.92) | 3.00 (0) |
| Girls (7) | | 3.71 (1.11) | 3.71 (0.95) |
| Second Grade | 7–8 | | |
| Boys (9) | | 3.22 (0.83) | 3.22 (0.44) |
| Girls (8) | | 3.13 (0.83) | 3.00 (0) |
| Third Grade | 8–9 | | |
| Boys (9) | | 2.78 (1.56) | 3.67 (1.00) |
| Girls (7) | | 2.71 (1.11) | 3.29 (0.76) |
| Fourth Grade | 9–10 | | |
| Boys (36) | | 3.03 (0.91) | 3.50 (0.77) |
| Girls (32) | | 2.94 (1.27) | 3.22 (0.79) |
| Fifth Grade | 10–11 | | |
| Boys (17) | | 2.88 (1.17) | 3.29 (1.05) |
| Girls (9) | | 3.33 (1.12) | 3.22 (0.67) |
| Sixth Grade | 11–12 | | |
| Boys (8) | | 2.88 (1.13) | 3.50 (0.93) |
| Girls (12) | | 3.33 (1.15) | 3.50 (1.00) |
| Seventh and Eighth Grades | 12–14 | | |
| Boys | | 2.48 (1.26) | 3.52 (0.92) |
| Girls | | 3.00 (1.10) | 3.29 (0.78) |
| Mean Score, Boys | | 2.70 | 3.39 |
| Mean Score, Girls | | 3.16 | 3.32 |

Table 9.3  Mean Scores (and Standard Deviations) for the SDT Emotional Content and Self-Image Scales in Responses by High School Students, Younger Adults, and Seniors

| Group | Emotional Content | Self-Image |
|---|---|---|
| High School Youths | | |
| Boys (45, 27) | 2.56 (1.31) | 3.41 (1.01) |
| Girls (49, 38) | 3.24 (1.22) | 3.42 (0.86) |
| Younger (average, 28.7 yrs) | | |
| Men (18) | 2.94 (1.41) | 3.61 (1.09) |
| Women (33) | 3.21 (1.17) | 3.24 (1.09) |
| Senior (average, 80.8 yrs) | | |
| Men (17) | 2.59 (1.28) | 3.71 (0.92) |
| Women (27) | 3.26 (1.20) | 3.15 (0.91) |

Table 9.4  Frequencies of Female Scores in the Emotional Content of Responses to the SDT Drawing from Imagination Task

| n | Age | Score | | | | |
|---|---|---|---|---|---|---|
| | | 1 | 2 | 3 | 4 | 5 |
| 44 Adults | 20–50 | 0 | 12 | 14 | 18 | 0 |
| 38 Adolescents | 16–19 | 2 | 9 | 4 | 14 | 9 |
| 32 Adolescents | 13–15 | 2 | 10 | 11 | 5 | 4 |
| 21 Girls | 10–12 | 0 | 5 | 9 | 2 | 5 |
| 32 Girls | 9–10 | 5 | 7 | 9 | 7 | 4 |
| 7 Girls | 8–9 | 0 | 4 | 2 | 0 | 1 |
| 8 Girls | 7–8 | 0 | 2 | 3 | 3 | 0 |
| 7 Girls | 6–7 | 0 | 1 | 2 | 2 | 2 |
| 189 | | 9 (5%) | 50 (26%) | 54 (29%) | 51 (27%) | 25 (13%) |

Table 9.5  Frequencies of Male Scores in the Emotional Content of Responses to the SDT Drawing from Imagination Task

| n | Age | Score | | | | |
|---|---|---|---|---|---|---|
| | | 1 | 2 | 3 | 4 | 5 |
| 18 Adults | 20–50 | 2 | 6 | 5 | 1 | 4 |
| 26 Adolescents | 16–19 | 5 | 7 | 10 | 0 | 4 |
| 34 Adolescents | 13–15 | 7 | 15 | 7 | 2 | 3 |
| 25 Boys | 10–12 | 5 | 2 | 12 | 4 | 2 |
| 36 Boys | 9–10 | 1 | 10 | 13 | 11 | 1 |
| 9 Boys | 8–9 | 3 | 1 | 1 | 3 | 1 |
| 7 Boys | 7–8 | 0 | 2 | 1 | 4 | 0 |
| 8 Boys | 6–7 | 5 | 1 | 2 | 0 | 0 |
| 163 | | 28 (17%) | 44 (27%) | 51 (31%) | 25 (15%) | 15 (9%) |

Table 9.6  Frequencies of Female Scores in the Self-Image of Responses to the SDT Drawing from Imagination Task

| n | Age | Score | | | | |
|---|---|---|---|---|---|---|
| | | 1 | 2 | 3 | 4 | 5 |
| 44 Adults | 20–50 | 0 | 1 | 43 | 0 | 0 |
| 38 Adolescents | 16–19 | 0 | 5 | 14 | 10 | 9 |
| 32 Adolescents | 13–15 | 0 | 2 | 18 | 19 | 3 |
| 21 Girls | 10–12 | 0 | 50 | 16 | 1 | 4 |
| 32 Girls | 9–10 | 1 | 1 | 22 | 4 | 4 |
| 7 Girls | 8–9 | 0 | 0 | 6 | 0 | 1 |
| 8 Girls | 7–8 | 0 | 0 | 8 | 0 | 0 |
| 7 Girls | 6–7 | 0 | 0 | 4 | 1 | 2 |
| 189 | | 1 (.5%) | 9 (5%) | 131 (69.5%) | 25 (13%) | 23 (12%) |

Table 9.7  Frequencies of Male Scores in the Self-Image of Responses to the SDT Drawing from Imagination Task

| n | Age | Score | | | | |
|---|---|---|---|---|---|---|
| | | 1 | 2 | 3 | 4 | 5 |
| 18 Adults | 20–50 | 0 | 4 | 6 | 1 | 7 |
| 26 Adolescents | 16–19 | 0 | 1 | 21 | 1 | 3 |
| 34 Adolescents | 13–15 | 1 | 0 | 13 | 13 | 7 |
| 25 Boys | 10–12 | 1 | 1 | 16 | 3 | 4 |
| 36 Boys | 9–10 | 0 | 1 | 21 | 9 | 5 |
| 9 Boys | 8–9 | 0 | 0 | 6 | 0 | 3 |
| 7 Boys | 7–8 | 0 | 0 | 5 | 2 | 0 |
| 8 Boys | 6–7 | 0 | 0 | 8 | 0 | 0 |
| 163 | | 2 (1.2%) | 7 (4.2%) | 96 (59%) | 29 (18%) | 29 (18%) |

**Table 9.8 Percentile Rank and *t*-Score Conversions for the STD Predictive Drawing Task**

| Grade | 1 | | 2 | | 3 | | 4 | | 5 | |
|---|---|---|---|---|---|---|---|---|---|---|
| Age | 6–7 | | 7–8 | | 8–9 | | 9–10 | | 10–11 | |
| Score | *t* | % | *t* | % | *t* | % | *t* | % | *t* | % |
| 1 | 36.26 | 4 | 24.67 | 1 | 22.10 | 1– | | | | |
| 2 | 36.91 | 10 | 28.67 | 2 | 25.86 | 1 | 24.00 | 1– | | |
| 3 | 41.55 | 15 | 32.67 | 4 | 29.63 | 2 | 27.86 | 1 | | |
| 4 | 46.20 | 35 | 36.67 | 9 | 33.40 | 5 | 31.72 | 3 | 24.90 | 1 |
| 5 | 50.84 | 53 | 40.67 | 18 | 37.16 | 10 | 35.58 | 7 | 29.46 | 2 |
| 6 | 55.49 | 71 | 44.67 | 30 | 40.93 | 18 | 39.44 | 14 | 34.02 | 5 |
| 7 | 60.14 | 84 | 48.67 | 45 | 44.70 | 30 | 43.30 | 25 | 38.57 | 13 |
| 8 | 64.78 | 93 | 52.68 | 61 | 48.46 | 44 | 47.16 | 39 | 43.13 | 25 |
| 9 | 69.43 | 97 | 56.68 | 75 | 52.23 | 59 | 51.02 | 54 | 47.69 | 41 |
| 10 | 74.08 | 99+ | 60.69 | 86 | 56.00 | 73 | 54.88 | 69 | 52.24 | 59 |
| 11 | | | 64.69 | 93 | 59.76 | 84 | 58.74 | 81 | 56.80 | 75 |
| 12 | | | 68.69 | 97 | 63.53 | 91 | 62.60 | 90 | 61.36 | 87 |
| 13 | | | 72.69 | 99+ | 67.30 | 96 | 66.46 | 95 | 65.91 | 94 |
| 14 | | | | | 71.06 | 98 | 70.32 | 98 | 70.47 | 98 |
| 15 | | | | | 74.83 | 99+ | 74.18 | 99+ | 75.03 | 99+ |

| Grade | 6 | | 7 | | 8 | | 10 | | adult | |
|---|---|---|---|---|---|---|---|---|---|---|
| Age | 11–12 | | 12–13 | | 13–14 | | 15–16 | | | |
| Score | *t* | % | *t* | % | *t* | % | *t* | % | *t* | % |
| 1 | | | | | | | | | | |
| 2 | | | | | | | | | | |
| 3 | 21.19 | 1– | | | | | 22.18 | 1– | | |
| 4 | 26.09 | 1 | 20.38 | 1– | | | 25.47 | 1 | | |
| 5 | 30.98 | 3 | 25.41 | 1 | | | 28.77 | 2 | | |
| 6 | 35.87 | 8 | 30.44 | 2 | 23.76 | 1– | 32.07 | 4 | 23.82 | 1– |
| 7 | 40.76 | 18 | 35.48 | 7 | 28.52 | 2 | 35.37 | 7 | 27.82 | 1 |
| 8 | 45.65 | 33 | 40.51 | 17 | 33.27 | 5 | 38.66 | 13 | 31.82 | 3 |
| 9 | 50.54 | 52 | 45.55 | 33 | 38.02 | 12 | 41.96 | 21 | 35.81 | 8 |
| 10 | 55.43 | 71 | 50.58 | 52 | 42.76 | 24 | 45.26 | 32 | 39.81 | 15 |
| 11 | 60.33 | 85 | 55.61 | 71 | 47.53 | 40 | 48.56 | 44 | 43.81 | 27 |
| 12 | 65.22 | 94 | 60.65 | 86 | 52.28 | 59 | 51.85 | 58 | 47.80 | 41 |
| 13 | 70.10 | 98 | 70.72 | 98 | 57.03 | 76 | 55.15 | 70 | 51.80 | 57 |
| 14 | 75.00 | 99+ | 75.75 | 99+ | 61.79 | 88 | 58.45 | 80 | 55.80 | 72 |
| 15 | | | | | 66.54 | 95 | 61.79 | 88 | 59.80 | 84 |

Table 9.9  Percentile Rank and *t*-Score Conversions for Drawing from Observation

| Grade | 1 | | 2 | | 3 | | 4 | | 5 | |
|---|---|---|---|---|---|---|---|---|---|---|
| Age | 6–7 | | 7–8 | | 8–9 | | 9–10 | | 10–11 | |
| Score | t | % | t | % | t | % | t | % | t | % |
| 1 | 28.84 | 2 | 29.83 | 2 | 22.32 | 1– | 28.51 | 2 | | |
| 2 | 32.85 | 4 | 32.88 | 4 | 25.78 | 1 | 31.60 | 3 | | |
| 3 | 36.86 | 10 | 35.94 | 8 | 29.24 | 2 | 34.69 | 6 | 23.76 | 1– |
| 4 | 40.87 | 18 | 38.99 | 14 | 32.70 | 4 | 37.78 | 11 | 27.88 | 1 |
| 5 | 44.89 | 30 | 42.05 | 21 | 36.16 | 8 | 40.87 | 18 | 32.00 | 4 |
| 6 | 48.91 | 46 | 45.11 | 31 | 39.62 | 15 | 43.96 | 27 | 36.12 | 8 |
| 7 | 52.92 | 61 | 51.22 | 55 | 43.08 | 25 | 47.05 | 38 | 40.24 | 16 |
| 8 | 56.93 | 75 | 54.27 | 67 | 46.54 | 36 | 50.15 | 51 | 44.36 | 29 |
| 9 | 60.95 | 86 | 57.33 | 77 | 50.00 | 50 | 53.24 | 63 | 48.48 | 44 |
| 10 | 64.96 | 93 | 60.38 | 85 | 53.46 | 64 | 56.33 | 74 | 52.60 | 60 |
| 11 | 68.97 | 97 | 63.44 | 91 | 56.92 | 75 | 59.42 | 83 | 56.72 | 75 |
| 12 | 72.99 | 99+ | 66.49 | 95 | 60.38 | 85 | 62.51 | 89 | 60.84 | 86 |
| 13 | | | 69.55 | 98 | 63.84 | 92 | 65.60 | 94 | 64.96 | 93 |
| 14 | | | 72.60 | 99+ | 67.30 | 96 | 68.69 | 97 | 69.08 | 97 |
| 15 | | | | | 70.76 | 98 | 71.78 | 99+ | 73.20 | 99+ |

| Grade | 6 | | 7 | | 8 | | 10 | | adult | |
|---|---|---|---|---|---|---|---|---|---|---|
| Age | 11–12 | | 12–13 | | 13–14 | | 15–16 | | | |
| Score | t | % | t | % | t | % | t | % | t | % |
| 1 | 24.53 | 1– | | | | | 34.57 | 6 | | |
| 2 | 27.52 | 1 | | | | | 36.51 | 9 | | |
| 3 | 30.51 | 3 | 23.68 | 1– | | | 38.46 | 13 | | |
| 4 | 33.50 | 5 | 27.47 | 1 | | | 40.40 | 17 | | |
| 5 | 36.49 | 9 | 31.25 | 3 | | | 42.35 | 22 | | |
| 6 | 39.48 | 15 | 35.03 | 7 | | | 44.29 | 28 | | |
| 7 | 42.47 | 23 | 38.81 | 13 | 23.32 | 1– | 46.23 | 35 | | |
| 8 | 45.46 | 33 | 42.59 | 23 | 28.41 | 2 | 48.18 | 43 | | |
| 9 | 48.45 | 44 | 46.37 | 36 | 33.50 | 5 | 50.12 | 50 | | |
| 10 | 51.44 | 56 | 50.15 | 51 | 38.59 | 13 | 52.07 | 58 | | |
| 11 | 54.43 | 67 | 53.93 | 65 | 43.69 | 26 | 54.01 | 66 | 17.79 | 1– |
| 12 | 57.42 | 77 | 57.71 | 78 | 48.78 | 45 | 55.95 | 73 | 27.40 | 1 |
| 13 | 60.41 | 85 | 61.49 | 87 | 53.87 | 65 | 57.95 | 79 | 37.02 | 10 |
| 14 | 63.40 | 91 | 65.27 | 94 | 58.96 | 82 | 59.84 | 84 | 46.63 | 37 |
| 15 | 66.39 | 95 | 69.05 | 97 | 64.05 | 92 | 61.79 | 88 | 56.25 | 74 |

| Grade | 1 | | 2 | | 3 | | 4 | | 5 | |
|---|---|---|---|---|---|---|---|---|---|---|
| Age | 6–7 | | 7–8 | | 8–9 | | 9–10 | | 10–11 | |
| Score | t | % | t | % | t | % | t | % | t | % |
| 1 | | | | | | | | | | |
| 2 | 24.79 | 1 | 23.36 | 1– | | | | | | |
| 3 | 29.30 | 2 | 27.38 | 1 | 24.20 | 1 | 22.35 | 1– | 22.23 | 1– |
| 4 | 33.81 | 5 | 31.40 | 3 | 28.79 | 2 | 26.39 | 1 | 26.66 | 1 |
| 5 | 38.32 | 12 | 35.41 | 7 | 33.38 | 5 | 30.43 | 2 | 31.08 | 3 |
| 6 | 42.83 | 24 | 39.43 | 14 | 37.97 | 12 | 34.48 | 6 | 35.50 | 7 |
| 7 | 47.34 | 39 | 43.45 | 25 | 42.56 | 23 | 38.52 | 13 | 39.93 | 16 |
| 8 | 51.84 | 57 | 47.46 | 40 | 47.15 | 39 | 42.56 | 23 | 44.35 | 28 |
| 9 | 56.35 | 74 | 51.48 | 56 | 51.74 | 57 | 46.61 | 37 | 48.77 | 45 |
| 10 | 60.86 | 86 | 55.50 | 71 | 56.33 | 74 | 50.65 | 53 | 53.20 | 63 |
| 11 | 65.37 | 94 | 59.52 | 83 | 60.92 | 86 | 54.69 | 68 | 57.62 | 78 |
| 12 | 69.88 | 98 | 63.53 | 91 | 65.51 | 94 | 58.74 | 81 | 62.05 | 89 |
| 13 | 74.38 | 99+ | 67.55 | 96 | 70.10 | 98 | 62.78 | 90 | 66.47 | 95 |
| 14 | | | 71.57 | 98 | 74.69 | 99+ | 66.82 | 95 | 70.89 | 98 |
| 15 | | | 75.59 | 99+ | | | 70.86 | 98 | 75.32 | 99+ |

| Grade | 6 | | 7 | | 8 | | 10 | | adult | |
|---|---|---|---|---|---|---|---|---|---|---|
| Age | 11–12 | | 12–13 | | 13–14 | | 15–16 | | | |
| Score | t | % | t | % | t | % | t | % | t | % |
| 1 | | | | | | | | | | |
| 2 | | | | | | | | | | |
| 3 | | | | | | | | | | |
| 4 | | | 21.75 | 1– | | | 24.36 | 1– | | |
| 5 | 23.84 | 1– | 25.54 | 1 | 21.80 | 1– | 27.66 | 1 | | |
| 6 | 29.00 | 2 | 29.33 | 2 | 26.29 | 1 | 30.97 | 3 | | |
| 7 | 34.15 | 6 | 33.11 | 5 | 30.78 | 3 | 34.28 | 6 | 23.03 | 1– |
| 8 | 39.31 | 14 | 36.90 | 10 | 35.27 | 7 | 37.59 | 11 | 27.93 | 1 |
| 9 | 44.46 | 29 | 40.68 | 18 | 39.76 | 15 | 40.90 | 18 | 32.84 | 4 |
| 10 | 49.62 | 48 | 44.47 | 29 | 44.25 | 28 | 44.21 | 28 | 37.74 | 11 |
| 11 | 54.77 | 68 | 48.25 | 43 | 48.74 | 44 | 47.52 | 40 | 42.64 | 23 |
| 12 | 59.93 | 84 | 52.04 | 58 | 53.23 | 63 | 50.83 | 53 | 47.55 | 40 |
| 13 | 65.08 | 93 | 55.82 | 72 | 57.72 | 78 | 54.14 | 66 | 52.45 | 60 |
| 14 | 70.23 | 98 | 59.61 | 83 | 62.21 | 89 | 57.45 | 77 | 57.36 | 77 |
| 15 | 75.39 | 99+ | 63.39 | 91 | 66.70 | 95 | 60.75 | 86 | 62.26 | 89 |

Table 9.10  Percentile Rank and t-Score Conversions for Drawing from Imagination

# The Silver Drawing Test and Draw a Story

| | Table 9.11 Percentile Rank and *t*-Score Conversions for SDT Total Scores | | | | | | | | | |
|---|---|---|---|---|---|---|---|---|---|---|
| Grade | 1 | | 2 | | 3 | | 4 | | 5 | |
| Age | 6–7 | | 7–8 | | 8–9 | | 9–10 | | 10–11 | |
| Score | *t* | % | *t* | % | *t* | % | *t* | % | *t* | % |
| 8 | 22.69 | 1– | 22.80 | 1– | | | | | | |
| 9 | 25.24 | 1 | 24.55 | 1 | | | | | | |
| 10 | 27.80 | 1 | 26.30 | 1 | | | | | | |
| 11 | 30.36 | 3 | 28.05 | 1 | | | | | | |
| 12 | 32.92 | 4 | 29.80 | 2 | | | 23.05 | 1– | | |
| 13 | 35.47 | 7 | 31.54 | 3 | 22.81 | 1– | 24.90 | 1 | | |
| 14 | 38.03 | 12 | 33.29 | 5 | 24.90 | 1 | 26.76 | 1 | | |
| 15 | 40.59 | 17 | 35.04 | 7 | 26.99 | 1 | 28.62 | 2 | 22.82 | 1– |
| 16 | 43.15 | 25 | 36.79 | 9 | 29.07 | 2 | 30.47 | 3 | 24.88 | 1 |
| 17 | 45.70 | 33 | 38.54 | 13 | 31.16 | 3 | 32.33 | 4 | 26.95 | 1 |
| 18 | 48.26 | 43 | 40.29 | 17 | 33.25 | 5 | 34.18 | 6 | 29.02 | 2 |
| 19 | 50.82 | 53 | 42.04 | 21 | 35.33 | 7 | 36.04 | 9 | 31.08 | 3 |
| 20 | 55.38 | 71 | 43.79 | 27 | 37.42 | 10 | 37.90 | 12 | 33.15 | 5 |
| 21 | 55.93 | 72 | 45.53 | 33 | 39.51 | 15 | 39.75 | 15 | 35.22 | 7 |
| 22 | 58.49 | 80 | 47.28 | 39 | 41.59 | 20 | 41.61 | 20 | 37.28 | 10 |
| 23 | 61.05 | 87 | 49.03 | 46 | 43.68 | 26 | 43.47 | 26 | 39.35 | 14 |
| 24 | 63.61 | 91 | 50.78 | 53 | 45.77 | 34 | 45.32 | 32 | 41.42 | 19 |
| 25 | 66.16 | 95 | 52.53 | 60 | 47.85 | 41 | 47.18 | 39 | 43.48 | 26 |
| 26 | 68.72 | 97 | 54.28 | 67 | 49.94 | 50 | 49.04 | 46 | 45.55 | 33 |
| 27 | 71.28 | 98 | 56.03 | 73 | 52.03 | 58 | 50.89 | 54 | 47.62 | 41 |
| 28 | 73.84 | 99 | 57.78 | 78 | 54.11 | 66 | 52.75 | 61 | 49.68 | 49 |
| 29 | 76.39 | 99+ | 59.52 | 83 | 56.20 | 73 | 54.61 | 68 | 51.75 | 57 |
| 30 | | | 61.57 | 87 | 58.29 | 80 | 56.46 | 74 | 53.82 | 65 |
| 31 | | | 63.02 | 90 | 60.37 | 85 | 58.32 | 80 | 55.88 | 72 |
| 32 | | | 64.77 | 93 | 62.46 | 89 | 60.18 | 85 | 57.95 | 79 |
| 33 | | | 66.52 | 95 | 64.54 | 93 | 62.03 | 88 | 60.02 | 84 |
| 34 | | | 68.27 | 97 | 66.63 | 95 | 63.89 | 91 | 62.08 | 89 |
| 35 | | | 70.02 | 98 | 68.72 | 97 | 65.75 | 94 | 64.15 | 92 |
| 36 | | | 71.77 | 99 | 70.80 | 98 | 67.60 | 96 | 66.22 | 95 |
| 37 | | | 73.51 | 99 | 72.89 | 99 | 69.46 | 97 | 68.28 | 97 |
| 38 | | | 75.26 | 99 | 74.98 | 99 | 71.31 | 98 | 70.35 | 98 |
| 39 | | | 77.01 | 99+ | 77.06 | 99+ | 73.17 | 99 | 72.42 | 99 |
| 40 | | | | | | | 75.03 | 99 | 74.48 | 99 |
| 41 | | | | | | | 76.88 | 99+ | 76.55 | 99+ |
| 42 | | | | | | | | | | |
| 43 | | | | | | | | | | |
| 44 | | | | | | | | | | |
| 45 | | | | | | | | | | |

*continued*

### Table 9.11 Percentile Rank and *t*-Score Conversions for SDT Total Scores (continued)

| Grade | 6 | | 7 | | 8 | | 10 | | adult | |
|---|---|---|---|---|---|---|---|---|---|---|
| Age | 11–12 | | 12–13 | | 13–14 | | 15–16 | | | |
|  | *t* | % | *t* | % | *t* | % | *t* | % | *t* | % |
| 8 | | | | | | | | | | |
| 9 | | | | | | | | | | |
| 10 | | | | | | | | | | |
| 11 | | | | | | | | | | |
| 12 | | | | | | | | | | |
| 13 | | | | | | | | | | |
| 14 | | | | | | | | | | |
| 15 | | | | | | | 26.49 | 1 | | |
| 16 | | | | | | | 27.86 | 1 | | |
| 17 | | | | | | | 29.23 | 2 | | |
| 18 | 24.94 | 1 | | | | | 30.61 | 3 | | |
| 19 | 27.33 | 1 | 26.96 | 1 | | | 31.98 | 4 | | |
| 20 | 29.72 | 2 | 28.83 | 2 | | | 31.35 | 5 | | |
| 21 | 32.11 | 4 | 30.71 | 3 | | | 34.73 | 6 | | |
| 22 | 34.50 | 6 | 32.58 | 4 | | | 36.10 | 8 | | |
| 23 | 36.89 | 10 | 34.45 | 6 | 24.96 | 1 | 37.47 | 11 | | |
| 24 | 39.28 | 14 | 36.32 | 9 | 27.04 | 1 | 38.84 | 13 | | |
| 25 | 41.68 | 20 | 38.19 | 12 | 29.12 | 2 | 40.22 | 16 | | |
| 26 | 44.07 | 28 | 40.07 | 16 | 31.20 | 3 | 41.59 | 20 | | |
| 27 | 46.46 | 36 | 41.94 | 21 | 33.28 | 5 | 42.96 | 24 | | |
| 28 | 48.85 | 45 | 43.81 | 27 | 35.36 | 7 | 44.34 | 28 | | |
| 29 | 51.24 | 55 | 45.68 | 33 | 37.44 | 10 | 45.71 | 33 | | |
| 30 | 53.63 | 64 | 47.55 | 40 | 39.52 | 15 | 47.08 | 39 | | |
| 31 | 56.02 | 73 | 49.42 | 48 | 41.60 | 20 | 48.46 | 44 | 27.50 | 1 |
| 32 | 58.41 | 80 | 51.30 | 55 | 43.68 | 26 | 49.83 | 50 | 30.18 | 2 |
| 33 | 60.80 | 86 | 53.17 | 63 | 45.76 | 34 | 51.20 | 55 | 32.86 | 4 |
| 34 | 63.20 | 91 | 55.04 | 69 | 47.84 | 41 | 52.57 | 60 | 35.54 | 7 |
| 35 | 65.59 | 94 | 56.91 | 75 | 49.92 | 50 | 53.95 | 66 | 38.21 | 12 |
| 36 | 67.98 | 96 | 58.78 | 81 | 52.00 | 58 | 55.32 | 70 | 40.89 | 18 |
| 37 | 70.37 | 98 | 60.65 | 86 | 54.08 | 66 | 56.69 | 75 | 43.57 | 26 |
| 38 | 72.76 | 99 | 62.53 | 89 | 56.16 | 73 | 58.07 | 79 | 46.25 | 35 |
| 39 | 75.15 | 99+ | 64.40 | 93 | 58.24 | 79 | 59.44 | 83 | 48.93 | 46 |
| 40 | | | 66.27 | 95 | 60.31 | 85 | 60.81 | 86 | 51.61 | 56 |
| 41 | | | 68.14 | 96 | 62.39 | 89 | 62.19 | 89 | 54.29 | 67 |
| 42 | | | 70.01 | 98 | 64.47 | 93 | 63.56 | 91 | 56.96 | 76 |
| 43 | | | 71.89 | 99 | 66.55 | 95 | 64.93 | 93 | 59.64 | 83 |
| 44 | | | 73.76 | 99 | 68.63 | 97 | 66.30 | 95 | 62.32 | 84 |
| 45 | | | 75.63 | 99+ | 70.71 | 98+ | 67.68 | 96+ | 65.00 | 93+ |

*Note:* The *t* scores are based on the unbiased estimate standard deviation. Percentile ranks are calculated from the table of cumulative normal probabilities, *Biometrika Tables for Statistics,* vol. 1, edited by E. S. Pearson and H. O. Hartley, and assume the scores are normally distributed. These procedures were used to avoid underestimating variability, because, for several grades, the population is small. —Beatrice J. Krauss, PhD

# Chapter 10

# Using the Silver Drawing Test with Clinical and Nonclinical Populations

◇    ◇    ◇

This chapter reviews studies that used the Silver Drawing Test (SDT) to assess the cognitive skills and attitudes of individuals and groups of children and adolescents with disabilities. It also compared their scores with the scores of those with no known impairments. Some studies examined the SDT performances of students with hearing impairments and learning disabilities as well as adolescents and adults with brain injuries; others examined age and gender differences in the spatial skills and attitudes of unimpaired children, adolescents, young adults, and senior adults.

## Cognitive Skills

### Comparing Hearing-Impaired and Hearing Students

The SDT was originally designed to tap the cognitive abilities of children like Charlie, who had such severe hearing and language impairments that the psychologist in his school declared his intelligence could not be tested. Nevertheless, he scored above the 90th percentile on the Torrance Test of Creative Thinking, as was discussed in chapter 6.

When Charlie was a young man, we met again at the reunion of exhibitors whose drawings and paintings were included in the Smithsonian Institution's traveling exhibition *Shout in Silence* and shown at the Metropolitan Museum of Art in 1976. He agreed to respond to the three drawing tasks that eventually became the SDT. Comparing his cognitive scores with those of typical, unimpaired adults, his 15 points in the Drawing from Imagination subtest—the maximum possible score—exceeded the adult norm or average of 12.64 points. In Drawing from Observation, he also scored 15 points, above the mean score of 13.88. His scores in Predictive Drawing cannot be compared with typical scores because at the time he took the test, only two of its three tasks had been developed. Nevertheless, Charlie received the maximum possible scores on the two tasks.

In expressing emotions, however, Charlie's score in Drawing from Imagination was below the norm, more negative: he scored 2 points on the emotional content scale, below the mean of 2.94 for young men. In self-image he scored 3 points, below the mean of 3.61, suggesting that Charlie's outlook was less optimistic and self-confident than that of typical young men his age. His responses are shown in figure 10.1.

Charlie's scores support the theory that the SDT scores of respondents with auditory or language impairments can equal the scores of unimpaired respondents. Additional support was provided by the findings of the State Urban Education Project (Silver, 1973), as was reported in chapter 6. In addition, Kopytin (2002) has found no significant differences between the scores of normal students and students with language impairments in Russia, as will be discussed in chapter

Figure 10.1a. Predictive Drawing by Charlie, age 24.

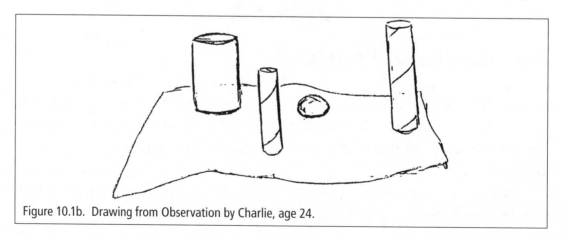

Figure 10.1b. Drawing from Observation by Charlie, age 24.

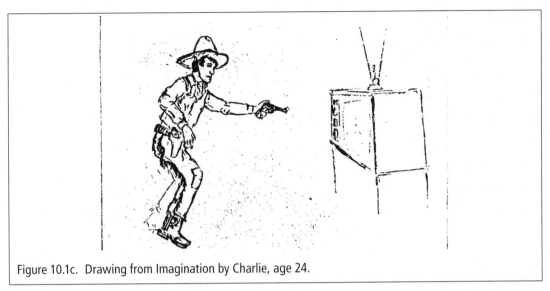

Figure 10.1c. Drawing from Imagination by Charlie, age 24.

12. Kopytin has concluded that the cognitive skills assessed by the SDT are independent of verbal skills. Subsequently, he has also found significant correlations between the SDT and the Torrance Test of Creative Thinking and other creativity tests, as was reported in chapter 8.

Recently, the SDT scores of 28 hearing children were compared with the scores of 27 deaf children, 13 girls and 14 boys, ages 9 to 11 in the fourth grade of a non-residential special school in New York City (Silver, 2002). One girl and one boy were severely impaired, not only with deafness but also with multiple handicaps; another boy had "language disorders." The hearing students included 14 girls and 14 boys attending two public elementary schools, matched in age and selected at random from responses to the SDT administered by a classroom teacher in New Jersey and an art therapist in Pennsylvania.

*Results*

In Predictive Drawing, no significant differences emerged between hearing and hearing-impaired students in horizontal orientation or ability to sequence. In vertical orientation, however, the deaf group received significantly higher scores ($F$ [1,51] = 14.34; $p < .001$). Mean scores were 3.13 and 2.00, respectively. No gender differences were found.

In Drawing from Observation, no significant differences were found between hearing and hearing-impaired students, nor between genders, in representing left/right, above/below, or front/back relationships.

In Drawing from Imagination, the hearing children received higher scores than the deaf children in ability to select ($F$ [1,51] = 12.85; $p < .001$), ability to combine ($F$ [1,51] = 57.66; $p < .000001$), and ability to represent ($F$ [1,51] = 30.99; $p < .000001$).

The girls received higher scores than the boys in ability to select (3.54 vs 3.04), to a degree significant at the .05 level ($F$ [1,51] = 5.49; $p < .05$).

*Observations*

Only 4 of the 55 children responded to the Predictive Drawing task by correctly drawing vertical houses on the slope, scoring 5 points, and 3 of these 4 were deaf. This finding suggests that they had become aware that houses remain vertical even on a slope, providing they are cantilevered or supported by posts. The finding was unexpected, because more than a few teachers, psychologists, and other highly educated adults have responded to the task incorrectly, drawing houses perpendicular to the slope, and receiving the lowest score of 1 point.

No significant differences were found in the four remaining spatial abilities, supporting the theory that children with hearing impairments can be expected to equal hearing children in the cognitive abilities measured by the Predictive Drawing and Drawing from Observation tasks of the SDT.

On the other hand, the deaf students had significantly lower scores in the Drawing from Imagination task, suggesting that selecting images and combining them into drawings may involve the same mental operations as selecting words and combining them into sentences. Perhaps language deficiencies tend to restrict experiences in selecting, combining, and representing. Would additional experiences through Drawing from Imagination enhance ability to select and combine words?

## Comparing Children with Hearing Impairments, Learning Disabilities, and No Known Disabilities

This study expanded the previous study by adding a sample of 28 children with learning disabilities. The data were analyzed to determine which groups differed on which measures.

The deaf children had higher scores in vertical orientation than did the children with learning disabilities and the unimpaired children to a degree significant at the .05 level of probability. No significant differences were found in sequencing or horizontality.

In Drawing from Observation, the children with learning disabilities had lower scores than the children who were deaf and those with no disabilities in representing left/right relationships. In representing above/below relationships, the unimpaired children scored higher than did the children with learning disabilities, and no significant differences between groups were found in representing front/back relationships.

The unimpaired students received higher scores in the abilities to select, combine, and represent than did the students with learning disabilities and those with hearing impairments. The girls received higher scores than did the boys in selecting and in combining; the boys received no higher scores in any of the abilities.

These findings support the theory that the SDT can be effective in assessing and comparing the cognitive strengths and weaknesses of girls and boys with hearing impairments, with learning disabilities, and without any disabilities.

## Clues to the Functioning of Patients with Brain Injuries

*Mr. O*

After suffering a cerebral hemorrhage, Mr. O, age 56, received therapy in a rehabilitation center (Silver, 2001). According to his speech therapist, he had both expressive and receptive language impairments. He spoke fluently but tended to confuse grammar and verb tenses, could not read aloud, and found it difficult to express concepts. He also had difficulty following a series of directions, such as "put the book on the table, and the pencil in your pocket." Asked to provide art therapy and assess his impairment, I used the SDT Drawing from Imagination task as a pre- and posttest in our first and last meetings.

Mr. O performed well in the Drawing from Observation and Predictive Drawing tasks, but in the Drawing from Imagination task he seemed confused. He selected stimulus drawings of a man and a woman, and then drew a series of stick figures and arrows to represent interaction between his subjects. This response scored 1 point each in the abilities to select, combine, and represent, and 3 points in emotional content (unemotional) and self-image (unclear).

At our second meeting, I presented Mr. O with the Form C stimulus drawings shown in chapter 13. He chose the mountain climber, and then drew "Gathering Magic Herbs" (fig. 10.2a), changing the mountain climber from a child to an adult with rope, axe, and flask. His climber had almost reached the top of the mountain, which was, perhaps, a metaphor for trying to recover from a stroke.

Mr. O then talked about the onset of his stroke. It began when he was having lunch with a friend, and he found himself unable to talk or even write. Nevertheless, he was aware of what was happening, and remained aware throughout his stay in the hospital.

At our last meeting, Mr. O responded again to the Drawing from Imagination task, choosing the cat and the snake and drawing "Hedges May Hide Surprises" (fig. 10.2b). The drawing may reflect anxiety about his plans to return to work the following day, but he offered no explanation, choosing to spend the rest of our meeting saying goodbye.

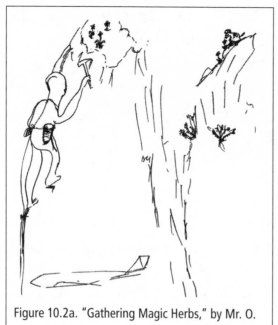

Figure 10.2a. "Gathering Magic Herbs," by Mr. O.

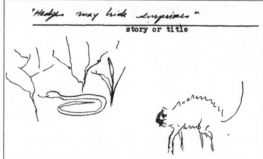

Figure 10.2b. "Hedges May Hide Surprises," by Mr. O—His Last Drawing from Imagination.

*Gary*

At age 15, Gary had suffered a stroke that left him unable to speak and paralyzed on both sides of his body, with movement limited to two fingers of his left hand. He could not sit unsupported, and because he had difficulty swallowing, he could not prevent saliva from escaping his mouth. He seemed to understand everything I said, however, and although he could not speak, he communicated by pointing to letters of the alphabet printed on a board in his lap. To signal the end of a word, he tapped the bottom of the board, as though it were the spacebar of a typewriter. Although he could not sit unsupported in his electric wheelchair, he maneuvered it skillfully, and responded to the drawing tasks with enthusiasm.

In Drawing from Observation with a felt-tipped pen held between his two functioning fingers, Gary included not only the cylinder arrangement, but also the table where it was placed, other objects on the table, and a nearby chair (see fig. 10.3a). This drawing revealed that he was able to perceive and represent spatial relationships in height, width, and depth, suggesting that his ability to draw from observation remained intact.

In the Drawing from Imagination task, Gary drew two cars, one above the other. Using the cartoon device of a balloon around the upper car to indicate that it was lower car's dream or fantasy, he also spelled out his title, "Dreaming About a Dune Buggy" (fig. 10.3b).

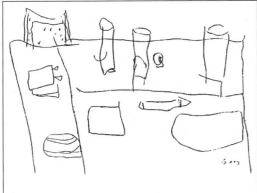

Figure 10.3a. Gary's Response to the SDT Drawing from Observation Task.

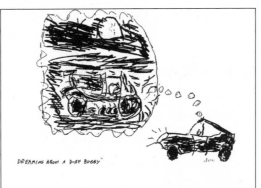

Figure 10.3b. Gary's Response to the SDT Drawing from Imagination Task "Dreaming about a Dune Buggy."

The idea of a car dreaming about another car suggests that Gary was alert and imaginative. The dreaming car, its headlights and taillights turned on, is green; the dreamed-about car is red, green's complementary color. Above it is the moon in dark sky, suggesting that the lower car, asleep and dreaming about its opposite, could symbolize Gary's immobility and yearning for romance.

Gary's ability to represent his thoughts through drawing from imagination also seemed intact.

Additional SDT responses by other patients with brain injuries are discussed elsewhere (Silver, 1975b; Sandburg, Silver, & Vilstrup, 1984; Silver, 2000a and 2000b).

# Age and Gender Differences

## Comparing Male and Female Adolescents

It is often assumed that males are superior to females in spatial ability. According to McGee (1979), psychological testing for more than 50 years has concluded that males consistently excel in spatial ability. It has even been claimed that male superiority in spatial thinking has been confirmed and is not in dispute (Moir & Jessel, 1992).

To test the assumption, responses to the Predictive Drawing and Drawing from Observation tasks from 33 girls and 33 boys (ages 12 to 15, attending public schools in Nebraska, New York, and Pennsylvania) were compared (Silver, 1996b).

No significant gender differences emerged. In representing depth, female mean scores (3.70) were higher than male mean scores (3.03), but the probability was less than .10 and did not reach significance. The girls received higher mean scores on four of the six tasks (horizontality, verticality, height, and depth), whereas the boys received higher mean scores in sequencing and horizontality (left/right relationships), but the differences did not reach significance. The boys' scores, like the girls' scores, tended to be consistent and did not show variability. These findings suggested that further investigation of gender differences would be worthwhile.

## Comparing Adults and Adolescents

A subsequent study asked if different scoring systems could explain why other investigators had found males superior to females in performing tasks designed to measure concepts of horizontality and verticality (Silver, 1998a). In search of answers, responses to the Predictive Drawing tasks by adults were added, and responses that previously had scored 5 points were scored again.

The subjects included 88 male and 88 female adolescents and adults. The adolescents included a class of college freshmen in Nebraska, a college audience in New York, and residents of a detention facility in Missouri. The adults included 26 men and 26 women, ages 18 to 50 (mean age, 26), who had participated in the previous study.

Once again, no significant gender differences were found, either in success-failure scores or in cognitive level scores. Chi-square analyses indicated that both males and females had lower scores in verticality than horizontality; males had lower verticality scores than females. The findings supported the previous study and suggested that perhaps some investigators had been assessing knowledge of physical phenomena rather than natural reference systems based on Euclidean concepts of space. The findings called into question the widespread assumption of male superiority in spatial intelligence and suggested that expressing spatial concepts nonverbally, through drawing, offers unique opportunities for assessing concepts of space. It also may be that self-confidence plays a critical role. Women tend to be less confident about the value of their ideas, and men tend to be more competitive.

These findings call into question the widespread assumption of male superiority in spatial intelligence. They also suggest that drawing offers unique opportunities to assess concepts of space. It also may be that self-confidence plays a crucial role. Women tend to be less self-confident, and men more competitive.

## Comparing Aging and Young Adults

Although much is known about aging adults in nursing homes, little is known about the cognitive skills of those who are psychologically, physically, and financially independent. This study compared the SDT scores of 57 aging and 51 young men and women (Silver, 1999, 2000c). The young adults attended colleges or participated in college audiences. The seniors, ages 64 to 95, lived independently in separate households and two retirement residences. Residence A provided many amenities, was relatively expensive, and provided lifetime care. Residence B provided fewer amenities and charged minimal fees. Three procedures were used to assess age and gender differences: individual responses, statistical analyses of mean scores, and top- and bottom-range scores.

Although no significant age differences were found when we compared the SDT performances of aging and young adults, surprising differences in scores emerged when we compared cognitive content, emotional content, self-image, and verticality, as shown in table 10.1 and figure 10.4.

Gender differences emerged to significant degrees. Men had higher scores in sequential order, horizontality, and self-image (portraying powerful or effective principal subjects more often). Both age groups followed similar patterns in emotional content, both peaking at the intermediate 3-point (ambiguous, ambivalent, or unemotional) level.

Drawings about unfortunate subjects or stressful relationships predominated in both age groups (32% seniors, 33% young adults), and less than 10% of either group drew sad individuals or life-threatening relationships (1 point).

Top- and bottom-range scores yielded information not found in the statistical analysis. A larger proportion of seniors than young adults received top scores in the ability to represent (55% and 41%, respectively). This trend was reversed for verticality in response to the Predictive Drawing task. More seniors drew vertical houses on the slope without providing adequate support (4 points), perhaps a metaphor for feeling unsteady on one's feet and reflecting an age-related change in the perception of verticality.

The unexpected finding of gender differences, not age differences, prompted a closer look at the performances of senior women. The 13 women in Residence A had higher mean scores than did the 13 women in Residence B, suggesting that dread of becoming incapacitated and forced into nursing homes may have affected the cognitive functioning of these residents. The findings suggested that being able to remain physically and financially independent could be a critical factor in successful aging.

Although no significant age differences were found when the SDT performances of aging and young adults were compared, surprising differences in scores emerged when comparing cognitive content, concepts of verticality, emotional content, and self images, as shown in figures 10.4 and 10.1.

To further analyze for potential age and gender differences in Predictive Drawing, the sample was expanded to include four age groups: 53 children, 66 adolescents, 36 seniors, and 51 young adults. Several age trends emerged.

For horizontality, there was a significant effect of age group ($F$ [1,196] = 18.61; $p < .0001$). Children (3.15) scored lower than adolescents did (4.17). Adolescents scored lower than did young adults (4.61), but did not differ from seniors (4.49). The young adults and senior adults did not differ.

# The Silver Drawing Test and Draw a Story

| | Older Adults | | | Younger Adults | | |
|---|---|---|---|---|---|---|
| **Table 10.1 Comparing SDT Performances of Older and Younger Adults** | | | | | | |
| | | *Drawing from Imagination* | | | | |
| | | *Emotional Content* | | | | |
| Score | *n* | % | Score | *n* | % | |
| 1 | 5 | 11% | 1 | 3 | 6% | |
| 2 | 13 | 30% | 2 | 17 | 33% | |
| 3 | 12 | 27% | 3 | 11 | 22% | |
| 4 | 6 | 14% | 4 | 11 | 22% | |
| 5 | 8 | 18% | 5 | 9 | 18% | |
| Total | 44 | | | 51 | | |
| | | *Self-Image* | | | | |
| Score | *n* | % | Score | *n* | % | |
| 1 | 1 | 2% | 1 | 1 | 2% | |
| 2 | 4 | 9% | 2 | 9 | 18% | |
| 3 | 27 | 61% | 3 | 23 | 45% | |
| 4 | 3 | 7% | 4 | 6 | 12% | |
| 5 | 9 | 20% | 5 | 12 | 24% | |
| Total | 44 | | | 51 | | |
| | | *Cognitive Content* | | | | |
| Score | *n* | % | Score | *n* | % | |
| 1 | 0 | 0 | 1 | 0 | 0 | |
| 2 | 0 | 0 | 2 | 0 | 0 | |
| 3 | 10 | 23% | 3 | 10 | 20% | |
| 4 | 9 | 20% | 4 | 20 | 39% | |
| 5 | 25 | 57% | 5 | 21 | 41% | |
| Total | 44 | | | 51 | | |
| | | *Predictive Drawing* | | | | |
| | | *Verticality* | | | | |
| Score | *n* | % | Score | *n* | % | |
| 1 | 2 | 6% | 1 | 2 | 5% | |
| 2 | 5 | 15% | 2 | 3 | 8% | |
| 3 | 10 | 29% | 3 | 5 | 14% | |
| 4 | 12 | 35% | 4 | 7 | 19% | |
| 5 | 5 | 15% | 5 | 20 | 54% | |
| Total | 34 | | | 37 | | |
| | | *Horizontality* | | | | |
| Score | *n* | % | Score | *n* | % | |
| 1 | 1 | 3% | 1 | 0 | 0 | |
| 2 | 0 | 0 | 2 | 0 | 0 | |
| 3 | 6 | 17% | 3 | 0 | 0 | |
| 4 | 8 | 23% | 4 | 11 | 29% | |
| 5 | 20 | 57% | 5 | 27 | 71% | |
| Total | 35 | | | 38 | | |

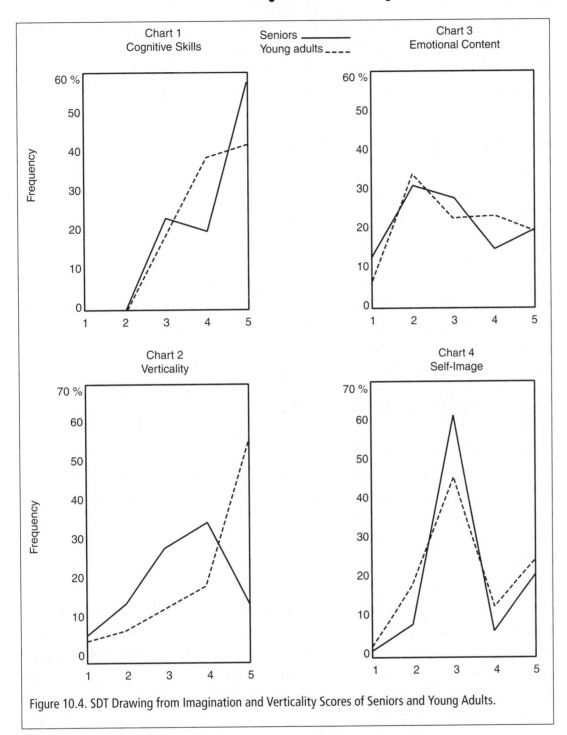

Figure 10.4. SDT Drawing from Imagination and Verticality Scores of Seniors and Young Adults.

For verticality, a main effect for age group emerged *(F* [1,197] = 12.30; *p* < .001). Children (1.98) scored lower than adolescents (2.64), who in turn scored lower than adults (3.53) and seniors (3.32). The adult groups did not differ.

For ability to sequence, there was a borderline significant effect *(F* [1,147] = 2.68; *p* < .10). Adolescents scored significantly higher than seniors did (4.52 vs 3.95).

Young adults scored in the middle (4.15) and did not differ from either group. Gender differences were also observed, but are not detailed here.

In general, it appears that there are few age-related changes in SDT performances. There may be a slight trend toward a decline in horizontality scores, but more study is needed to test this hypothesis.

### Hiscox's Study of Students with Learning Disabilities

Hiscox (1990) administered the SDT and the California Achievement Test to 14 children with learning disabilities, 14 with dyslexia, and 14 children with no known disabilities in the third, fourth, and fifth grades of three public schools and one private school in California. An examination of reliability showed a high level of interscorer agreement; ratings varied by only 1 to 3 points. Using a one-way analysis of variance, Hiscox found that each group performed differently. On both tests, normal subjects had the highest mean scores. The subjects with learning disabilities had higher mean scores than the subjects with reading disabilities who performed within the middle range of both groups. The results supported her hypothesis that children with learning disabilities would fall within the normal range.

### Henn's Study of Students with Multiple Disabilities

Henn (1990) used the SDT Drawing from Observation task as a pre- and posttest measure of whether an integrated approach to teaching can have a significant effect on the understanding of spatial relationships by students with multiple disabilities. Subjects included 24 racially mixed retarded students (ages 16 to 21) from rural, suburban, and urban areas in three New York counties. Some students were nonverbal. Henn devised six lesson plans to develop spatial awareness and elicit spatial thinking with movement activity accompanied by music and art. Scoring was done blindly by Henn and another certified art teacher whose interscorer reliability coefficients were .95 for horizontal relationships, .86 for vertical relationships, and .84 for depth. In addition, a correlation of .92 was found for combined gains on the three variables. The posttest scores for all three criteria we significantly higher than pretest scores. The combined pretest mean was 7.88 and the combined posttest mean 14.12, suggesting that the teaching approach enhanced understanding of the three spatial concepts to a highly significant degree, and that the SDT was effective as a pre- and posttest measure.

### Marshall's Study of Students with Learning Disabilities

Marshall (1988) used the SDT as both pre- and posttest to assess the effectiveness of a developmental program designed to enhance the cognitive skills of two groups of children with learning disabilities (ages 7 to 10 and ages 13 and 14) in the special education program of a school in Maine. The program included stimulus drawings, painting, modeling clay, drawing from observation, and playing "imagination games." After the program, the mean scores of the younger group increased in each task (with the most marked and consistent increase being in Drawing from Imagination), their total mean increasing from 16.24 to 21.09. The adolescent group showed little gain, their mean score increasing from 25.50 to 26.0.

# Attitudes

## Attitudes toward Self and Others

A preliminary study asked whether children tend to draw fantasies about subjects who were of the same gender as themselves (Silver, 1992). It examined responses to the SDT Drawing from Imagination task by 145 boys and 116 girls (ages 7 to 10), second, third, and fourth graders in suburban and urban public schools in Nebraska, New Jersey, New York, and Pennsylvania, as well as Canada. Highly significant gender differences emerged: most boys drew pictures about male subjects, girls, about female subjects.

A subsequent study asked if there were significant differences in ages and attitudes, as well as choosing same-gender subjects (Silver, 1993a). The subjects included 531 subjects in five age groups: children, ages 7 to 10; younger adolescents, ages 13 to 16; older adolescents, ages 17 to 19; younger adults, ages 20 to 50; and older adults, ages 65 and over.

Males expressed positive attitudes toward solitary subjects and negative attitudes toward relationships. These differences were significant at the .001 level of probability ($A^2 = 46.971$; $p < .001$). Females expressed positive attitudes toward solitary subjects and both positive and negative attitudes toward relationships. These findings, too, were significant at the .001 level of probability ($A^2 = 25.32$; $p < .001$).

Males showed a significantly higher frequency than females in drawings about assaultive relationships ($A^2$ [1] $= 9.38$; $p < .01$). However, age and gender differences interacted ($A^2$ [4] $= 13.07$; $p < .05$), resulting in a significant age variability in assaultiveness for females but not for males. The proportion of older females who drew assaultive fantasies exceeded the proportion of older men who did so, as well as exceeding the proportion of all other female age groups.

The converse age and gender interaction was found for caring relationships ($A^2$ [4] $= 12.52$; $p < .05$). Females showed a significantly higher frequency of caring relationships across age groups; males showed significant age variability. The proportion of younger men who drew caring relationships exceeded the proportion of younger women, as well as exceeding the proportion of all other male age groups.

Respondents who drew human subjects chose subjects the same gender as themselves to a degree significant at the .001 level of probability. This tendency peaked in childhood and reached its lowest level among adults. The decline continued among older women (19%), but reversed among older men (54%), a proportion almost equal to that found in the samples of boys. Genders were clearly indicated in responses by children and adolescents, but were sometimes unclear in responses by adults—particularly in the drawings of older women.

## Attitudes toward the Opposite Sex

Early studies had found that respondents tend to draw positive fantasies about subjects the same gender as themselves, but negative fantasies about the opposite sex (Silver, 1992, 1993a). A subsequent study asked whether drawings about the opposite sex expressed negative attitudes to a significant degree (Silver, 1997a, 2001).

Reviewing responses to the Drawing from Imagination task from 480 children, adolescents, and adults, the study found that approximately one of four respondents (116) drew principal subjects of the opposite sex (21% males, 27% females). The responses were divided into age and gender groups, and mean scores analyzed.

The study included 222 male and 258 females, children, adolescents, and adults. The children, ages 8 to 11, attended six elementary schools in New Jersey and New York. The adolescents, ages 12 to 19 and in grades 7 through 12 and freshmen in college, resided in Nebraska, New York, Ohio, and Pennsylvania. The younger adults, ages 20 to 50, included older college students and residents of Nebraska, New York, and Wisconsin. The senior adults, ages 65 and older, lived independently in New York and Florida.

Several age and gender trends emerged, showing an age difference of borderline significance. Opposite-sex drawings increased with age from 29% of the children to 44% of the adolescents, and 77% of the adults. The remaining subjects chose animal subjects or subjects the same gender as themselves. There was no interaction.

The children and adolescents were more negative toward subjects of the opposite sex than were the adults ($F$ [1,112] = 2.77; $p$ < .10). For example, a girl, age 7, chose the stimulus drawing of the bride and the bed, then drew a sad-looking bride with what appears to be a dark bruise on one cheek, holding a dinner tray (presumably intended for the groom) who was lying in bed. Although the title is noncommittal, the drawing suggests domestic abuse.

"The Lady Getting Married to a Dog Who Wants to Kill Him" was an ambiguous but negative response by a boy, age 8, who chose the bride and the knife.

With snakes in her veil, the bride holds the knife in one hand, a bouquet in the other.

More males than females drew fantasies about the opposite sex. Both genders expressed more negative than positive feelings toward their subjects of the opposite sex, peaking at moderately negative (2 points), with most portraying them as ridiculous.

Although an analysis of variance found that males expressed significantly more negative feelings toward females than did females toward males, at the .01 level of significance ($F$ [1,112] = 6.92; $p < .01$), they were not necessarily expressing misogyny. If it is typical to project self-image through drawings, then drawings about opposite-sex subjects are likely to symbolize the other, not the self. It would seem to follow that feelings of superiority or disgust could be expected in drawings about others, just as drawings about the self tend to elicit positive associations, as studies have found.

It is important to remember that only 21% of the males and 27% of the females in this study drew subjects of the opposite sex. It may be that unhappy experiences were triggered by the stimulus drawings they chose and associated with their fantasies. The findings suggest that drawings about opposite-sex subjects could provide access to conflicts or troubling relationships, and thereby, opportunities for clinical discussion.

## Attitudes toward Food or Eating

Of the 15 stimulus drawings in Form A of the SDT, only two represent food or eating (the ice cream soda and the refrigerator), and both seem to trigger associations with feeling deprived. For example, a male adolescent selected the soda and drew "Not Having." It shows two young men standing side by side; one scowls, the other smiles. The scowling man is empty handed; the smiling man holds an ice cream soda, blackened for emphasis. An elderly woman chose two stimulus drawings, the refrigerator and the bride. In her drawing "Food for Thought. Does Marriage Fill a Void?" the bride kneels before the refrigerator, its open door revealing only two items of food.

Other responses seem ambivalent rather than negative. A woman who chose the soda and the girl drew "I Tell Her Not to Eat Sugar Then I Do" (fig. 10.5). A young girl, age 9, chose the same stimulus drawings, and then drew "A Sneaky Snacker" (fig. 10.6); the girl's expression and posture suggest guilty desire. Another nine-year-old girl chose the soda and the mouse, drawing the soda too tall for the mouse to reach.

Since these and other drawings suggest that choosing the soda or refrigerator might serve to identify respondents with eating disorders, the responses of 293 children, adolescents, and adults were reexamined (Silver, 1998b).

The children, ages 9 to 10, attended fourth grade in three elementary schools in New Jersey, New York, and Pennsylvania. The younger adolescents, ages 12 to 15,

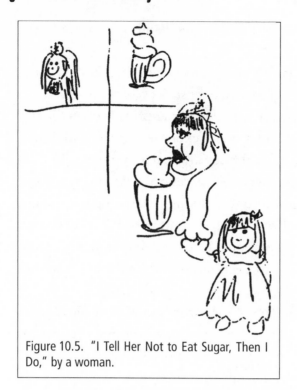

Figure 10.5. "I Tell Her Not to Eat Sugar, Then I Do," by a woman.

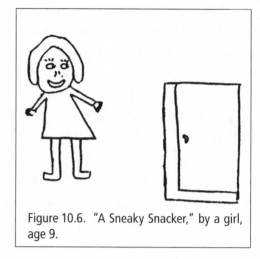

Figure 10.6. "A Sneaky Snacker," by a girl, age 9.

attended grades 7 to 10 in five public schools in Nebraska, New York, and Pennsylvania. The older adolescents, ages 16 to 18, included high school seniors in two public high schools in New York. The adults, ages 19 to 70, included a class of college students in Nebraska; adults in college audiences in Idaho, New York, and Wisconsin; and older adults in Florida.

Almost one-third of the 293 respondents (29%) and more than twice as many females (59 females, 26 males) drew fantasies about food or eating—proportionally more females than males in each of the four age groups. Among females, these drawings included almost half of the older adolescents, ages 16 to 18 (46.9%), about one-third of the younger girls (34.4%), and more than one-fourth of the women (27.9%). Among males, the largest proportions again appeared in the sample of younger adolescents ages 13 to 15 (29.4%) and boys ages 9 to 10 (25%), followed by adolescents ages 16 to 18 (22.2%), and ending with the sample of men (10%).

Another notable gender difference was found in responses that were ambivalent, ambiguous, or unclear: 45% of the women and girls, compared with 23% of the men and boys, scored 3 points.

Because adolescent girls tend to be particularly vulnerable to eating disorders, and the sample of older adolescent girls in this study drew proportionally more fantasies about eating than did other age or gender groups, further investigation might determine whether the SDT can be useful in identifying those whose preoccupations might be undetected or masked.

## The Attitudes of Older Adults

A subsequent study expanded the previous study by examining more closely the responses of 59 adults over the age of 65: 28 men and 31 women living independently in their communities (Silver, 1993b). Although the sample was too small for statistical analysis, more older women than any other age or gender group drew sad or helpless solitary subjects (1 point). On the other hand, more older women than any other age or gender group drew pictures about active solitary pleasures (5 points).

In drawings about relationships, more older men than older women or any other age or gender group drew fantasies about stressful relationships (2 points). Older men expressed attitudes toward relationships that were proportionally more negative than those of any other male age group. Older women expressed more negative attitudes toward solitary subjects than those of any other age or gender group. Although negative attitudes predominated among older adults, they also used humor more often than did any other age group. Humor was used more often in responses by older men (39%) than in responses by older women (16%). The humor of adolescents tended to be aggressive, making fun of others, whereas the humor of older adults tended to be self-disparaging, directed toward themselves, perhaps reflecting resilience in spite of low self-esteem and the ability (or wish) to survive in spite of adversity.

# Section III

# The Use of Both Assessments by Practitioners in Florida and Abroad

◇    ◇    ◇

# Chapter 11

# Use of the Silver Drawing Test and Draw a Story by Art Therapists in the Miami-Dade County Public Schools in Florida

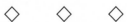

## Overview by Linda Jo Pfeiffer, EdD, ATR-BC

During the 2000–2001 school year, the Clinical Art Therapy Department in the Miami-Dade County Public Schools (M–DCPS) adopted the Silver Drawing Test of Emotion and Cognition (SDT) as an assessment tool to use with students identified as emotionally handicapped or severely emotionally disturbed. The district supported the adoption of the SDT by providing training in the form of in-service workshops and by purchasing *Art as Language* (Silver, 2001) for each of the 20 art therapists employed by M–DCPS.

The SDT is one of the two district-approved art therapy assessments. Since M–DCPS art therapists function within the learning environment of a school, the SDT is an invaluable tool offering a pre- and posttest modality that fits well within the education system. Each student on the art therapist's roster is assessed before beginning art therapy. From gathered information and the assessment tool, a report is developed and written (see our Form A, below). The art therapist collaborates with the student's teachers and other professional staff members to formulate and record goals and benchmarks on the student's individual education plan (IEP). Students receive individual or small group art therapy one time per week in sessions lasting anywhere from 30 to 60 minutes. At the close of each student's IEP year, the student is reassessed using the same assessment tool (see form B, below).

The SDT has been very useful in providing measurable outcomes. The pre- and posttest aspects of the SDT lend the test well to documenting positive gains or losses. It provides an alternative to traditional school testing by highlighting the student's previously undetected strengths. These strengths often include spatial intelligence, creativity, and the ability to select and combine images. It is also an indicator of cognitive weaknesses. The Drawing from Imagination task is especially helpful in deciphering aggressive tendencies, depression, tangential thinking, and fantasy on one spectrum and groundedness, sequential thinking, and creativity on another.

For children who are often overwhelmed emotionally, the SDT provides a familiar structure and the routine of paper and pencil. It provides a framework and level of comfort for children who have difficulty communicating verbally and helps them process concepts and arrange their thoughts in a comprehensive manner.

In addition to the SDT, M–DCPS art therapists implement the Draw a Story (DAS) assessment when a student has scored 1 point on the Emotional Content Scale and 1 point on the Self-Image Scale, or 1 point on the Emotional Content Scale and 5 points on the Self-Image Scale, as measured by the Drawing from Imagination task of the SDT. The DAS assessment is administered to determine if the student's emotional lability needs to be immediately addressed by the team (see form C, below). With the violence currently being perpetuated by students against other students, and the increase of adolescent suicide, the DAS may serve as a forewarning of potentially dangerous behaviors in children.

To illustrate how art therapists working within the schools are employing the SDT and DAS, we use the following forms to record case histories. By acquiring information about a student's level of cognitive functioning and emotional well-being, art therapists are able to design treatment plans that meet individual needs.

Form A
Miami-Dade County Public Schools
DIVISION OF EXCEPTIONAL STUDENT EDUCATION
CLINICAL ART THERAPY ASSESSMENT REPORT

NAME: _____ DOB: _____ ID#: _____ DATE: _____

ASSESSMENT: Silver Drawing Test of Cognition and Emotion (SDT)

SCHOOL:_____ ART THERAPIST: _____

REASON FOR ASSESSMENT

The SDT was conducted to ascertain if this student may benefit from art therapy as a mode of remediation and intervention, to compare emotional and cognitive functioning levels with the normative population, and to develop goals to help this student access education.

CLINICAL HISTORY

Brief description of significant historical data and documentation of sources of historical information. See Procedures Handbook.

PROCEDURE

The Silver Drawing Test of Cognition and Emotion (SDT) was administered. The SDT includes three tasks: Predictive Drawing, Drawing from Observation, and Drawing from Imagination. The SDT has two components, cognitive and emotional. Used in this assessment were an SDT test booklet, setup materials, and a pencil with an eraser. During the assessment, this therapist observed the student at work and, after he or she finished drawing, posed scripted and nonscripted questions.

SUMMARY OUTCOME

Focus on what is relevant. Do not reiterate what is found in the checked off box below. If humor is seen in the drawings, make sure you reference it here and comment on how it was used.

# The Silver Drawing Test and Draw a Story

Form B

Miami-Dade County Public Schools

DIVISION OF EXCEPTIONAL STUDENT EDUCATION

CLINICAL ART THERAPY PROGRESS REPORT

NAME: _____ DOB: _____ ID#: _____ DATE: _____

ASSESSMENT: Silver Drawing Test of Cognition and Emotion (SDT)

SCHOOL:_____ ART THERAPIST: _____

The following information represents this student's progress in art therapy during the school year, from _____ to_____ . This student attended *(write inidivdual or group and for how many minutes per week)*. *(He or she made or did not make)* positive strides toward meeting his or her goals as outlined in the PEN(s) of his or her current IEP.

*(Write a short paragraph describing the student's behaviors.)*

*(Write a short paragraph describing the student's themes in art therapy.)*

The Silver Drawing Test of Cognition and Emotion (SDT) was readministered and compared with the SDT results obtained *(write date of initial SDT)* (see chart below).

The student *(has made improvements, has not made improvements, has stayed the same)* in the areas of Emotional Content, Self-Image, and Drawing from Observation. His or her initial SDT portrayed themes that were *(state the themes)*. His or her posttest portrayed themes that were *(state the themes)*. *(Write what results this implies.)*

| Pretest | Scale/Task | Posttest | Normative Data | Above the Mean | Average/at the Mean | Below the Mean |
|---------|-----------|----------|----------------|----------------|---------------------|----------------|
| 2.5 | Emotional Content | | | | | |
| 2.5 | Self-Image | | | | | |
| N/A | Use of Humor | | | | | |
| 8 | Drawing from Imagination | | | | | |
| 12 | Predictive Drawing | | | | | |
| 5 | Drawing from Observation | | | | | |

Based on these findings and teacher reports, *(this student appears to need, not need non-traditional forms of counseling to access his or her education)*. It is recommended that *(write your recommendations for the student's new IEP)*.

## TEST RESULTS FROM THE SDT

| Scale/Task | Pretest | Normative Data | Above the Mean | Average/at the Mean | Below the Mean |
|---|---|---|---|---|---|
| Emotional Content | | | | | |
| Self-image | | | | | |
| Use of Humor | | | | | |
| Drawing from Imagination | | | | | |
| Predictive Drawing | | | | | |
| Drawing from Observation | | | | | |

The following recommendations are suggested as a result of the SDT.

## RECOMMENDATIONS

(*In this area write recommendations that are based upon your findings and correlate with the student's Priority Educational Needs (PENs). Give teachers recommendation on how they might best approach this child educationally given your findings about personality, learning style, self-esteem, emotional and cognitive functioning.*)

Form C

Miami-Dade County Public Schools

DIVISION OF EXCEPTIONAL STUDENT EDUCATION

CLINICAL ART THERAPY

Addendum to the Silver Drawing Test of Emotion and Cognition (SDT)

NAME: _____ DOB: _____ ID#: _____ DATE: _____

ADDENDUM ASSESSMENT: Draw a Story Assessment (DAS)

SCHOOL: _____ ART THERAPIST: _____

## RATIONALE FOR ADMINISTRATION

The Draw a Story Assessment (DAS) is administered to those students whose scores in the SDT Drawing from Imagination task indicated that picture stimuli of a more emotive nature might elicit responses that are highly correlated with depression and aggression.

*(It is suggested that you administer the DAS when a student's scores from the initial SDT Drawing from Imagination are one of the following:*

*A score of 1 point in both self-image and emotional content*

*A score of 5 points in self-image and 1 point in emotional content*

*A score of 1 point in the use of humor)*

## PROCEDURE

Used in this assessment were a DAS test booklet and a pencil with an eraser. The DAS assessment, like the SDT Drawing from Imagination task, asks respondents to choose two subjects from an array of stimulus drawings (Form A), imagine something happening between the subjects they choose, and then show what is happening in drawings of their own. When the drawings are finished, stories are added and discussed whenever possible and responses are scored on a 5-point rating scale (Silver, *Three Art Assessments*, 2002).

## SUMMARY OUTCOME

*(You are looking for whether or not there is a consistency in emotional states and attitudes toward the self. Discuss consistency if there is one. Focus on the theme (humor, self-image, emotional content) presented by the student. Compare the DAS response to the SDT Drawing from Imagination task. Consistently negative themes may be indicative of a precarious emotional state.)*

## RECOMMENDATIONS

*(If you base your goals and recommendations both the SDT and DAS be sure to state so.)*

# Mark and Lanette by Melinda Fedorko, ATR-BC

## Mark

Mark was a 10-year-old boy starting fourth grade when he began art therapy. He had many issues to cope with at home, including parental divorce due to domestic violence; his mother's recent bout with cancer, which was in remission; and his own health problems with asthma. He entered special education classes due to short attention span, aggression, leaving the class without permission, refusal to do work, and depression.

His first response to the SDT Drawing from Imagination task in August 2004 clearly reflects his parent's situation. The mother snake is warning the rat not to come near the baby snakes and the two eggs in the nest (see fig. 11.1a.). Mark must have also felt some separation from his mother (perhaps due to her illness), as he stated that the snake lived in another tree; however, he drew her in the same tree in order to protect her offspring.

Five months later, after art therapy began, Mark was improving in school and in therapy. Home life was still difficult—both parents were in new relationships and Mark was estranged from his father. Again, in his response (to the DAS assessment) he seems to mirror his home situation by drawing a dinosaur and a snake fighting (see fig. 11.1b). The tree, representing Mark, is directly in the middle of the snake

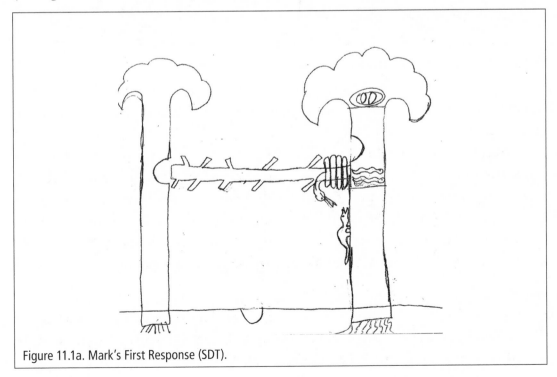

Figure 11.1a. Mark's First Response (SDT).

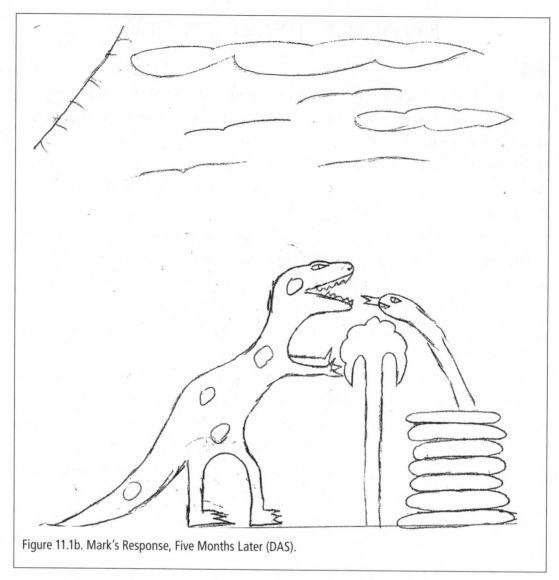

Figure 11.1b. Mark's Response, Five Months Later (DAS).

and dinosaur, as if he is trying to mediate the situation. The dinosaur eats the snake in the story.

Sixteen months after treatment began, Mark drew his latest response for the DAS assessment (see fig. 11.1c). In this elaborate picture he appears to be the dinosaur. A volcano exploding and a castle are off in the distance. In his story, the dinosaur wants to save his favorite tree, as he sees that lava balls are going to hit it. He decides to run to the safety of the castle. It appears as if Mark has found his solution by symbolically leaving the chaos of home and finding security outside of the family.

## Lanette

Lanette was 12 years old when she began art therapy. Her symptoms included aggression, audiovisual hallucinations, and an eating disorder, and she was in the school's special education program. When she responded to the drawing task for the first

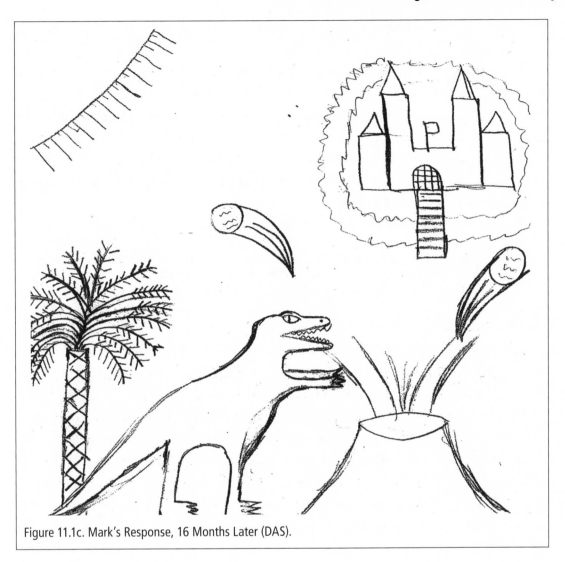

Figure 11.1c. Mark's Response, 16 Months Later (DAS).

time, she chose two stimulus drawings from SDT Form A, the cat and the mouse, but changed them in her drawing. The stimulus drawing cat scowls and the mouse smiles, standing upright, its tail down. In Lanette's drawing, however, only the cat smiles; the mouse is horizontal, its tail up, and between them, she wrote, "men, men, men" (see fig. 11.2a). Lanette's story was "The cat is chase [*sic*] the rat. The story I'm talking about is the food chain." Since the relationship seems stressful for the mouse, her drawing scored 2 points on the Emotional Content Scale and, since Lanette seems to identify with her mouse, 2 points on the Self-Image Scale.

In her second response—the DAS assessment—Lanette chose the girl and the snake. In her drawing, the bride has no arms or hands and the snake's head is at her groin. As she dictated, "There was a girl and a snake and the snake was attacking her and she said, 'Help me!'" (see fig. 11.2b). This drawing about a life-threatening relationship in which Lanette seems to identify with the victim scored 1 point in both emotional content and self-image. Both drawings seem to indirectly represent sexual abuse.

Responding to the DAS assessment two months later, Lanette again chose the cat and mouse, but this time her mouse was upright, and her cat no longer smiled. As she dictated, "The cat is chasing the rat and the rat ran inside its home. The cat couldn't get him so he waited outside for the rat but it didn't come out no more" (see fig. 11.2c). In her drawing, however, the mouse is no closer to home and safety than it is to the cat and danger. Since her drawing seems to contradict her words, it scored 3 points in both emotional content and self-image.

Eighteen months after her first response, she drew a fourth response:

> One day there was a mouse and a refrigerator. He went to go get some food to eat and a man walked into the kitchen and saw the mouse and the mouse ran back into his home. So the man had some people to get all the mices out of his home [see fig. 11.2d].

Near the bottom of her sketch she added, "Thank you for helping me." It is not clear whether the man is thanking the exterminator for helping him get rid of vermin or whether Lanette is indirectly expressing thanks. Her drawing is no longer about helpless victims, but about a subject who solves a problem effectively, with professional assistance, and scores 3.5 points in both emotional content and self-image.

I lost contact with Lanette when she entered the sixth grade, but recently, following my request, the art therapist at her school administered the DAS assessment to Lanette again. This time Lanette drew a smiling stick figure with an open parachute passing over sharp mountain peaks and an erupting volcano. At first glance, this seems alarming, and perhaps Lanette could again be in danger. However, she wrote, "The story is about a man is [*sic*] over a volcano. Who is going to see what's happening. He find a hill and rocks." When asked for further information by the art therapist Lanette stated, "He's an explorer" (see fig. 11.2e).

As seen through her SDT and DAS drawings, Lanette has continued to exhibit emotional growth and self-confidence. While her environment may seem treacherous or difficult (sharp peaks and a volcano), Lanette no longer sees herself as a victim—being chased or in hiding—but as an independent explorer.

This is a developmentally appropriate drawing. Although still a special education student, Lanette is again taking mainstream classes and is doing well. The SDT and DAS were helpful in diagnosing and monitoring her therapeutic progress.

## Peter by Enid Shayna Garber, ATR-BC

Peter is currently 11½ years old. During his two years in art therapy he has had many issues to deal with at home, including rejection by his father and stepfather, his moth-

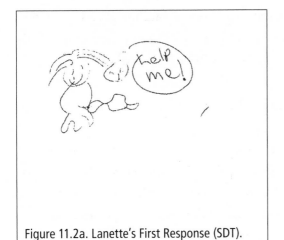

Figure 11.2a. Lanette's First Response (SDT).

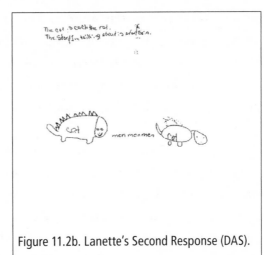

Figure 11.2b. Lanette's Second Response (DAS).

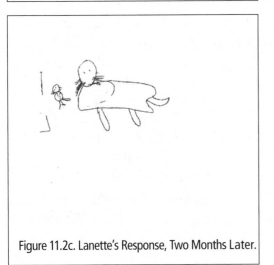

Figure 11.2c. Lanette's Response, Two Months Later.

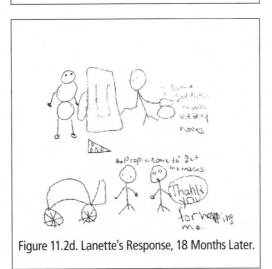

Figure 11.2d. Lanette's Response, 18 Months Later.

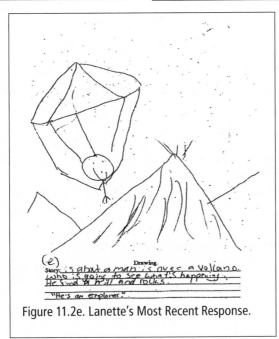

Figure 11.2e. Lanette's Most Recent Response.

er's divorce from his stepfather, and the recent death of his biological father. Peter's biological sister was recently in the custody of her biological father. Peter's mother has overcompensated for Peter's losses and emotional wounds, and as a result Peter is extremely dependent on adults, unmotivated, and insecure. Peter was referred to special education classes due to aggression toward others and a lack of academic gains in general education.

The initial SDT was administrated to determine emotional levels of functioning in order to formulate an art therapy treatment plan. Although the entire SDT was administered, this section focuses on the Drawing from Imagination task because it provided the most insight into Peter's emotional issues. Peter responded fully to the opportunity to use the structure of the stimulus drawings to bring issues from the unconscious into the present. The results of the initial Drawing from Imagination task were a starting point for addressing Peter's issues in art therapy treatment. The second SDT was administered to correlate with the updating of Peter's annual individual education plan (IEP) and to update goals for art therapy treatment. The third SDT was administered one year later to correlate with the updating of Peter's IEP and art therapy goals. I now have three results from the Drawing from Imagination task with which to identify changes with regard to an ongoing theme of getting needs met.

Peter's initial selection of the two subjects, a cat and a mouse, was repeated in the two reassessments that followed the initial assessment. The changes in Peter's reactions to how his subjects related to each other provided insight into the symbolic meaning of Peter's emotional life. Each story illustrated what Peter himself was unaware of on a conscious level. The theme of these three drawings pointed to the symbolic expression of succeeding in getting one's needs met, moving from magical thinking to being resourceful when faced with obstacles, and, finally, to independence and self-reliance.

Peter's initial drawing from imagination was "The Noticeable Cat" (see fig. 11.3a):

> The mouse got a little hungry. He smelled a big block of cheese and then the mouse went out of the hole and the cat saw him come out. The mouse did not know the cat saw him. Then the mouse sees the cat coming to him, so he jumped to the cheese. He reached the edge of the shelf. He got the cheese and ran to his hole as fast as he could. The cat tried to get him but he couldn't. He tried and tried but he couldn't.

Peter said that he identified with the mouse because he won. Symbolically, the tiny mouse outwits the cat with his magical ability and accomplishes the impossible.

Peter's second drawing from imagination was "The Mouse That Wants the Cheese" (see fig. 11.3b):

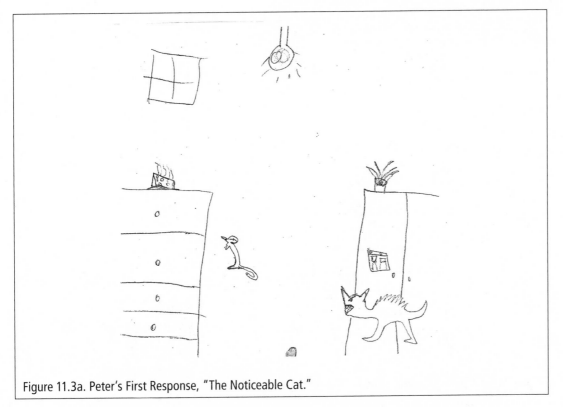

Figure 11.3a. Peter's First Response, "The Noticeable Cat."

One day a mouse was getting hungry and then peeked out to see if the coast was clear. At the time, nobody was in the kitchen. He spotted the cheese but it was very high up [an obstacle] but he saw a chair [resourceful] right next to the cheese. When he climbed the chair a lady spotted the mouse [another obstacle] going for the cheese and brought her cat with her [a third obstacle]. She put her cat down and found a stool and stood on it so the mouse could not get her. The mouse's friend [dependency, rescue, resourceful] appears and puts a web on the lady's mouth so she can't scream. The mouse gets the cheese and distracts [resourceful] the cat so he [the mouse] can get away.

Peter's third drawing from imagination is shown in figure 11.3c. In this story the mouse gets the cheese; however, when he runs to the safety of his hole, he makes it to safety—but without the cheese. Symbolically, this was a startling change in Peter's ability to meet his needs. By giving up the cheese he is learning to accept that he has had to make difficult choices in order to succeed. In this story Peter is accepting the responsibility that comes with independence.

In each story, Peter identified with the mouse that, although tiny and vulnerable, reaches safety. The progression seen from each assessment to the next speaks to the changes that Peter was experiencing in trying to reach his goals.

The goal in art therapy treatment is to help Peter develop a realistic approach to functioning independently. Peter needs to recognize that obstacles are a reality of life

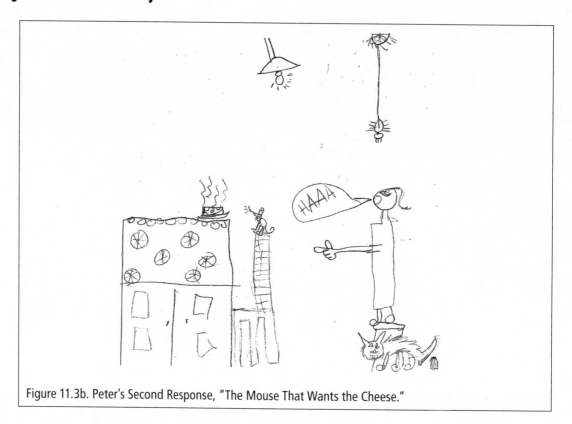

Figure 11.3b. Peter's Second Response, "The Mouse That Wants the Cheese."

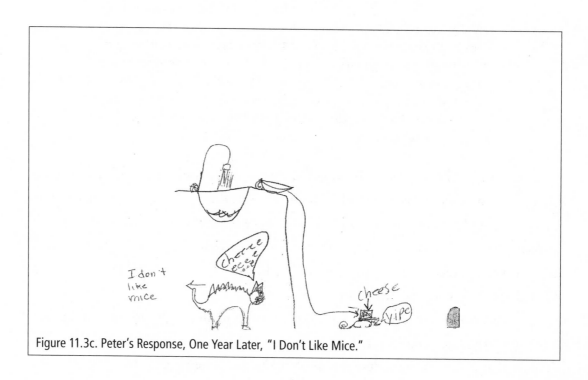

Figure 11.3c. Peter's Response, One Year Later, "I Don't Like Mice."

for everyone, and that he can remove the obstacle he puts in his path by believing he is worthy of happiness and success.

## Julio, Treatment Planning, and the SDT by Jennifer Blackmore, ATR-BC

Julio is a sixth grader in a program for severely emotionally disturbed students. Prior to this placement he was in a hospital homebound program as a result of his refusal to attend school due to the extreme emotional and physical reaction this would cause. In October 2003 he was hospitalized for anxiety and depression. His emotional difficulties are the result of significant traumas, including exposure to domestic violence between his parents, homelessness, and the loss of his grandfather.

I administered the SDT to determine whether art therapy would be an appropriate intervention for Julio, and to design a treatment plan that would help him succeed in the general curriculum. His overall score was average or above average in all areas, with the exception of self-image and the scores of the Drawing from Imagination task. In the abilities to select, combine, and represent he scored 3 points. He chose several stimulus drawings and drew "My Day" (see fig. 11.4a). It depicts a typical day for him, playing his PS2 video game, eating, and going to sleep, interrupted by his dog chasing an oversized rat that is eating the family's food. Julio's smiling self stands in sharp contrast to this disturbing environment.

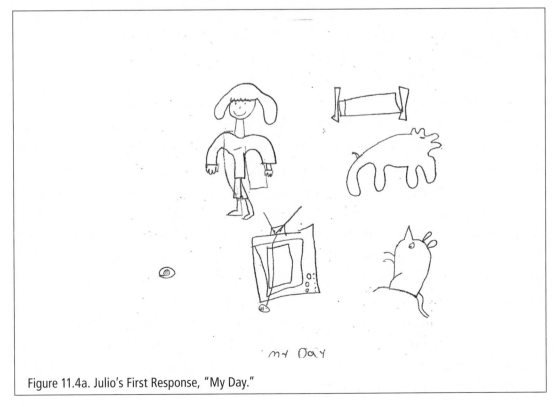

Figure 11.4a. Julio's First Response, "My Day."

His score of 3 out of 5 points on the Self-Image Scale was below average, and suggested a perception that was ill defined, ambivalent, and passive. He seemed to be an observer in his environment, accepting reality, however stressful and dangerous. This was his way of coping with aspects of his life, both past and present, over which he had little or no control.

The results of this test were consistent with other testing. Academically, he struggles with reading comprehension. As a result of these findings, therapeutic goals focused on strengthening his self-image, increasing his expression of feelings, and developing associative thinking skills.

For several months in art therapy, Julio worked on a multimedia sculpture using a wide range of materials. The sculpture was a symbol of his vision of an ideal home in the future where he lived happily with his two best friends. In the middle of his sculpture home he constructed a wishing well (so that all of their wishes would come true). The process of creating this artwork elicited myriad thoughts and feelings about traumatic events in his life, worries about the future, and fears about his basic needs not being met.

The protective environment of art therapy gave Julio an opportunity to resolve conflicts relating to his past, gain a healthier perspective on his life, and begin to look ahead to a promising future. I encouraged him to make associations, both cognitively and emotionally, among all of the elements in his imagined environment. Julio was proud of his inventiveness and adeptness with the media. He created a home that was well organized, a home that brought him happiness and security. Symbolically, it was rich and inviting; guardian angels watched over all of the inhabitants. It gave him hope.

Julio's progress in art therapy coincided with increased stability at home and success in the school setting. He seemed to feel more confident, and more connected and secure, in both places. At school he made the honor roll, was involved in schoolwide activities, and was developing meaningful friendships. At home, family stressors seemed to have abated, and he received praise and recognition from both parents for his academic success.

The SDT was readministered following six months of treatment. Results of the posttest indicated both emotional and cognitive gains. Julio's scores on the Self-Image and Emotional Content Scales increased from 3 to 5 points. In Drawing from Imagination, his scores improved as well, from 3 to 5 points in abilities to select and represent. He again chose several stimulus drawings and drew a family scene in which his father instructs his sister to turn off the TV and do her homework (see fig. 11.4b). He placed himself beside her, helping her. The image suggests family structure, support, and stability. The results of the SDT substantiate Julio's progress. The information gleaned from the SDT was invaluable in developing a highly focused and effective treatment plan for Julio.

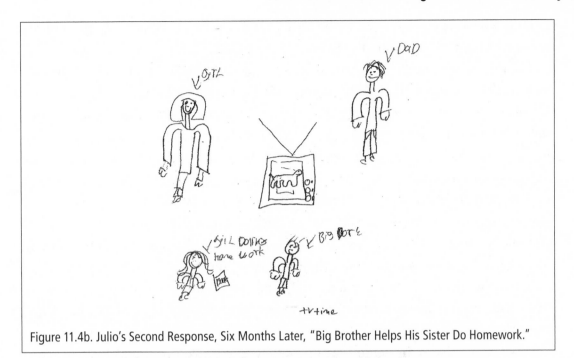

Figure 11.4b. Julio's Second Response, Six Months Later, "Big Brother Helps His Sister Do Homework."

## The SDT and DAS as Tools for Interdisciplinary Treatment Planning by Raquel Farrell-Kirk, ATR-BC

Art therapists have access to information about a student's level of functioning that is not readily available to other disciplines and treatment team members. Communicating clinical conceptualizations in a clear and concise manner can be accomplished through the use of an assessment tool such as the Silver Drawing Test (SDT) and the Draw a Story (DAS) assessment.

In my experience as an art therapist I have found that the SDT and DAS both provide an effective format for communicating important clinical concerns to other disciplines. These assessments are concise and therefore easy to administer and score in preparation for interdisciplinary team meetings. The availability of quantitative scores and norms for comparison make them more user friendly for other disciplines. The DAS and the Drawing from Imagination task of the SDT both illustrate key emotional issues in a succinct manner. The following case demonstrates the pivotal role that SDT and DAS results play in illuminating treatment issues and impacting treatment planning.

Mathew, a white male, is a seventh grader in the emotionally handicapped program of a large urban middle school. Little social history is available. He currently resides with his biological mother and his younger sister. His school records indicate a history of several years of disruptive behavior, impulsive actions, and defiance of school authority. His work style during both psychological evaluations and classroom assignments has been characterized as careless and impulsive. Testing reports indicate an average IQ, but below-grade-level academic performance.

I administered the SDT as part of the intake process for art therapy. Mathew's drawing from imagination, "The Princess Who Couldn't Laugh" (see fig. 11.5a), describes a king who summons people to try to make his daughter laugh. When someone finally does make her laugh, she laughs so hard that she has difficulty breathing and dies. The theme seems to represent Mathew's ambivalence about establishing interpersonal relationships and honestly displaying emotion. Although he said the story was based on a movie, it resembles a Norwegian fairy tale about a princess who was very serious and would never smile. In the fairy tale, there is a happy ending as an unlikely suitor is able to make the princess laugh. He is rewarded with her hand in marriage and half the kingdom and they, of course, live happily ever after. Mathew's use of this story may indicate that he lacks the confidence to create his own drawing and story. That he selected this particular tale to recreate suggests that he identifies with its emotional theme. His story lacks a happy ending, leaving one with the impression that displaying emotions openly, even positive ones, will have negative consequences.

Last year, Mathew was accused of writing a "hit list" that included both students and staff, but he denied being the author. At the time of the incident he admitted to suicidal ideation though he denied intent or plan. Subsequently, his mother was called, but she was nonresponsive. His stepfather was called to the school for a conference with the assistant principal. It was recommended that the student receive mental health services in the community. He received a suspension for his alleged involvement in the hit list.

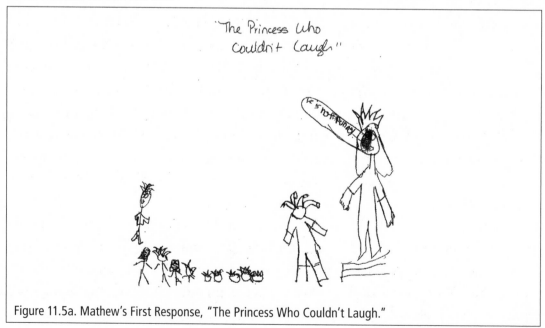

Figure 11.5a. Mathew's First Response, "The Princess Who Couldn't Laugh."

In the middle of the current school year, Mathew was referred to the school psychologist for an evaluation. The school psychologist, who had not met him before, conducted a complete battery of tests and gathered information from the teachers and clinical staff. Mathew's projective tests yielded only that he was guarded and appeared depressed. However, Mathew's recent work in art therapy raised concerns regarding his potential for violence. His most recent project involved a reproduction of the mask associated with a pop-culture horror movie icon. When asked to discuss his associations to this mask, he initially denied any attraction to the violence associated with the movies. After further discussion, he indicated some rationalization in his way of thinking about violence. In his opinion, whether or not harming another person is right or wrong depends on whether or not anyone else cares about the victim. He denied any specific thoughts of harming anyone.

The DAS assessment was administered at the next session to screen for signs of depression and potential aggression. The drawing was completed hastily with little attention to detail. He stated as he began the drawing, "I'm not even trying," and sat slumped in the chair, leaning back away from the paper as he drew. He drew a volcano, which he explained explodes and melts a nearby castle (see fig. 11.5b). The violence and destruction of this theme are countered by his story, which indicates that the princess in the castle ran away to escape harm and warned all other inhabitants to escape as well. He also stated that the castle was later rebuilt. When asked who or what in the picture he identified with he chose the volcano, which he described as "out of control."

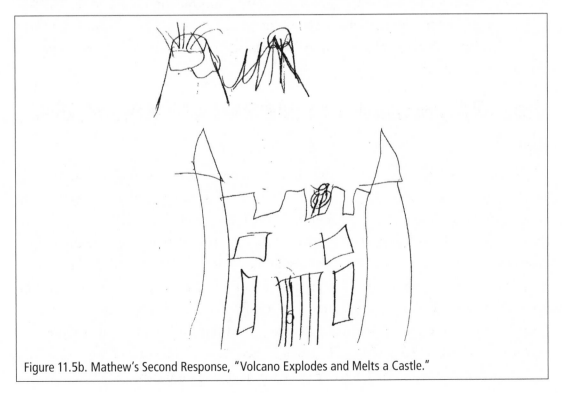

Figure 11.5b. Mathew's Second Response, "Volcano Explodes and Melts a Castle."

## The Silver Drawing Test and Draw a Story

There is a consistent theme of ambivalence across Mathew's drawing from imagination from the SDT and his DAS. His drawing from imagination seems to indicate ambivalence about both interpersonal relationships and displaying emotions. The current DAS indicates ambivalence about violent or destructive acts.

Mathew's conflicted feelings surrounding interpersonal relationships can make it difficult for him to establish trust in others. He appears to be on his own to manage his "out of control" emotions. Viewed in context of his history of defiant behaviors, suicidal ideation, and alleged involvement in the hit list, his violent imagery becomes even more alarming.

The SDT and DAS provided a way for me to share emotional themes in Mathew's artwork with the school psychologist and others in a concise and easily interpreted format. As a result, they were able to see that there was indeed cause for concern. The information regarding Mathew's emotional state was not revealed in the psychological testing administered. Without the opportunity for nonverbal expression and the stimulus drawings of the DAS, I do not believe this student's inner state would have been communicated.

Unfortunately, one week after sharing my concerns about the potential for escalating behaviors, Mathew was referred to administration for raising his hand as if to strike a teacher. Though he did not hit the teacher, this was considered a serious offense, and when compared to his previous infractions represented a clear escalation of violent behavior for him. An interdisciplinary team meeting is scheduled to discuss Mathew's academic and behavioral problems and explore possible placement in a more restrictive educational program with more intensive clinical services, including continued art therapy.

## Mario and Hispanic Students in the United States by Cheryl Earwood, ATR-BC

### Mario

A 17-year-old student in April 2004, Mario was raised in a strictly fundamentalist religious home, where his father, a pastor, was quite dominating. His father had recently divorced Mario's biological mother and then married another woman within three months. Mario had been diagnosed with attention deficit disorder; behavioral problems; and schizophrenia, chronic paranoid type. Testing revealed a full-scale IQ of 87. Some of his remarks indicated obsession with violent and sexual behavior toward females. He was banned from one teacher's class for a semester because she felt threatened by these remarks. Hitting, kicking, and refusing to obey rules were also reported. In therapy, he expressed fear that he would lose control and hurt someone, but felt that it would be the fault of the victim if that should happen. In responding to the SDT Drawing from Imagination task, he chose the dog and cat, and drew the fantasy "The Dog Is Barking at the Cat and the Cat Got Scared and Arched Its Back and Got Stifed" (see fig. 11.6a). After writing his title, Mario said, "Sometimes cats will run away and find a tree, but I'm afraid this one was killed."

A year later, in April 2005, Mario was able to relate his artwork to himself and his feelings, and it had become increasingly positive. He was more able to communicate in his counseling and art therapy sessions, there were no fights, and referrals for bizarre comments made in class had decreased considerably. He attended three classes a day, which reduced his anxiety, and appeared ready to increase the time he spent in school. Responding to the drawing task again, Mario chose the snake and mouse, then drew figure 11.6b. His story was:

> The snake is going after the mouse. She plans to eat him. The mouse has two little weapons and a helmet, and is determined to stand up to her saying, 'I won't let you kill anymore mice.' The mouse is able to defend himself.

His score in emotional content increased from 1 to 3.5 points, and in self-image from 3 to 3.5 points.

This reassessment drawing suggested progress in both the emotional and self-image domains. His response now contained humor and positive expectations for overcoming a threatening situation rather than expectations that lethal violence would occur. The outcome changed to one of survival.

By March 15, 2006, Mario was able to create positive artwork in response to assignments, draw problematic situations in his life, and symbolize and identify feelings in his artwork. He chose the stimulus drawing of the dog and the bug, then drew figure 11.6c. His smiling dog says, "What are you doing, little bug?" The bug

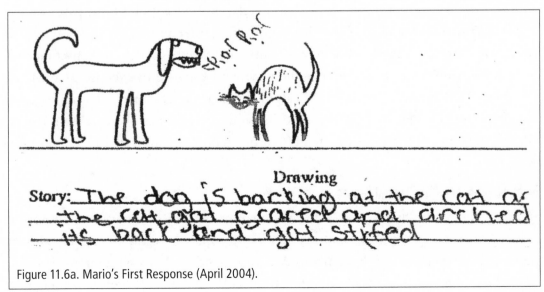

Figure 11.6a. Mario's First Response (April 2004).

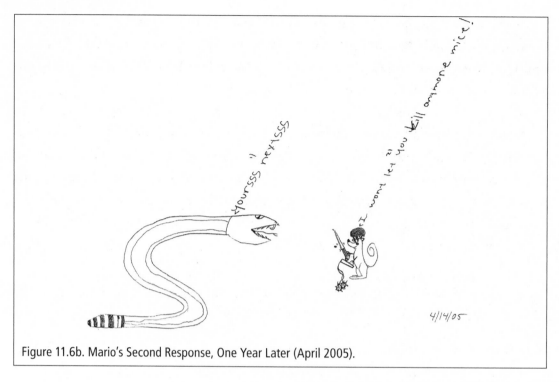

Figure 11.6b. Mario's Second Response, One Year Later (April 2005).

responds, "I won't be squashed!" The perception now is that the dog means no harm and the bug's assertiveness removes it from a dangerous situation without the need for fighting or violence, scoring 3.5 points in self-image and 4 points in emotional content.

Mario's cognitive scores in the abilities to select, combine, and represent increased from the 18th percentile in 2004 to the 66th percentile in 2006. His score in predictive drawing declined from the 80th to the 70th percentile, and his score in drawing from observation increased from the 79th to the 84th percentile.

In school, he was able to develop trusting relationships with both the psychologist and the art therapist, and his father joined him for a therapy session to resolve some issues. He currently attends school for the entire day. He has successfully participated on a sports team, won a district championship, and engaged in exercise each day of the week. He has not taken any medication this year. There have been no fights or inappropriate behavior toward girls, and his only problem has been arriving late to school, and an unwillingness to attend Saturday school as required for students who are tardy.

## Hispanic Students in the United States

In a previous study (Silver, 2002), Earwood compared Hispanic with non-Hispanic students in the Miami-Dade County school system, where 52.8% of the student population is Hispanic, 33% is African American, and 14.2% is white non-Hispanic or "other." Approximately 58% of the students do not have English as their pri-

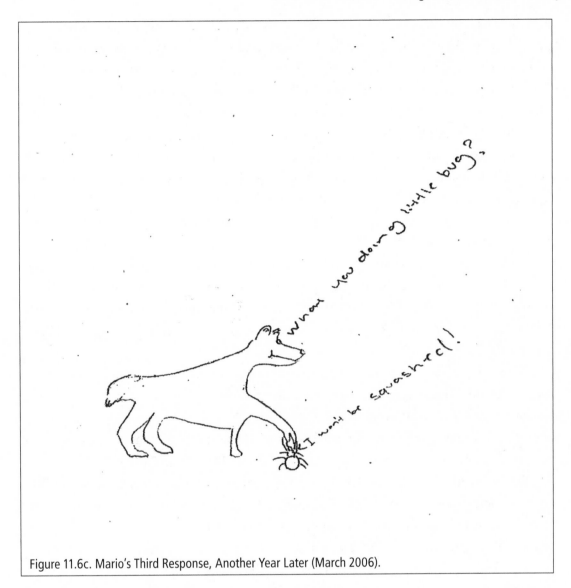

Figure 11.6c. Mario's Third Response, Another Year Later (March 2006).

mary language, and more than 59% of the district's students are eligible for free and reduced lunch.

Earwood administered the SDT to 30 students, ages 14 to 16 (20 boys and 10 girls), from a class in English for speakers of other languages. Previously, they had resided in South or Central America; they had been in the United States less than one year. Their responses were compared with the responses of 30 students of approximately the same ages, attending public schools in Indiana, Pennsylvania, and suburban and urban New York.

The total scores did not reveal much, but when the scores were examined separately, differences between groups emerged. In total self-image scores, 53% of the

Hispanic students, compared with 47% of the U.S. control group, responded with positive themes; 6%, compared with 13%, responded with negative themes, and 33%, compared with 47%, with ambiguous, ambivalent, or unemotional themes.

When positive self-image scores were examined separately, substantially more Hispanic students scored 5 points, seeming to identify with subjects who were powerful, loved, destructive, assaultive, or achieving goals (40% Hispanic, 27% controls). On the other hand, fewer Hispanic than U.S.-born adolescents drew moderately positive self-images, seeming to identify with subjects portrayed as fortunate but passive scored 4 points (13% Hispanic, 20% controls).

When negative self-image scores were examined separately, more than three times as many Hispanic students seemed to identify with subjects portrayed as frightened, frustrated, or unfortunate, scoring 2 points (10% Hispanic, 3% controls). Small but equivalent proportions of both groups (3%) seemed to identify with subjects portrayed as sad, isolated, or in mortal danger, scoring 1 point. Although their numbers tend to be few, any student who draws a strongly negative self-image warrants attention.

When negative emotional content scores were examined separately, more than twice as many Hispanic students scored 1 point, drawing pictures about violent relationships or sad, isolated individuals (23% Hispanic, 10% controls). At 2 points, however, the findings reversed: substantially fewer Hispanic than controls drew stressful relationships or unfortunate solitary subjects (20% Hispanic, 37% controls).

When positive emotional content scores were examined separately, fewer Hispanic students scored 4 points (13% Hispanic, 17% controls), drawing fantasies about friendly relationships or fortunate solitary subjects, but more scored 5 points, drawing loving relationships or effective solitary subjects (20% Hispanic, 17% controls).

The finding that 40% of the Hispanic adolescents, compared with 27% of U.S.-born adolescents, scored 5 points on the Self-Image Scale suggests that the Hispanic adolescents were feeling more secure and confident in themselves. Although separated from their native countries less than one year, they did not seem to be experiencing acculturation stress, as measured by responses to the SDT. The fact that they resided in Miami, within a large population of Spanish-speaking residents, may have played a critical role.

This finding accords with the finding of two large studies that compared the prevalence of psychiatric disorders among Mexican immigrants and U.S.-born residents. Vega et al. (1998) examined 3,012 adults of Mexican origin in California and found that 24% had experienced 12 of the disorders listed in the American Psychiatric Association's *Diagnostic and Statistical Manual of Mental Disorders*, third edition, compared with 48.1% of U.S.-born respondents. They concluded that despite very low education and income levels, Mexican Americans had lower rates of lifetime psychiatric disorders compared with rates reported for the U.S. population, and that psychiatric morbidity among Mexican Americans is primarily influenced by cultural variance rather than socioeconomic status. Mexican immigrants in the United States had lifetime rates similar to those of citizens of Mexico, whereas rates for Mexican American citizens were similar to those in the United States.

Escobar (1998) has found that immigrants, compared with patients born in the United States, had significantly lower prevalence of depression and posttraumatic stress disorder, despite their lower socioeconomic status. As Dr. Pfeiffer observed, it may be that an expansive sense of family contributes to the positive SDT responses of Spanish-speaking students in Miami. Extended families such as distant cousins and three or four generations may be more likely than small families to engender feelings of security and confidence, suggesting that by widening our circle of shared experiences, we gain mutual support and extend the boundary between "us and them."

# Chapter 12

# Use of the Silver Drawing Test and Draw a Story by Practitioners Abroad

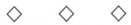

This chapter asks whether responses to the Silver Drawing Test (SDT) and Draw a Story (DAS) reveal cultural differences and similarities among respondents in Australia, Brazil, Russia, Thailand, and the United States, and whether the assessments are relatively free from cultural bias.

## Russia

### The Silver Drawing Test

Kopytin and Svistovskaya recently have found significant correlations between scores in ability to represent in the SDT Drawing from Imagination task, and scores on the Torrance Test of Creative Thinking (Torrance, 1984) as well as the Creativity Assessment Packet (Williams, 1980), as was reported in chapter 8.

Previously, Kopytin, a psychiatrist and art therapist, had translated the SDT and conducted a normative study with the assistance of 11 psychologists in Russia who collected samples and administered the tasks. They sent the response drawings to Kopytin, who scored and analyzed them with the assistance of a psychologist skilled in statistical analysis (Kopytin, 2002).

# The Silver Drawing Test and Draw a Story

Subjects of this normative study included 702 children, adolescents, and adults in large cities and small towns in various parts of the Russian Federation. The children and adolescents included 350 girls and 294 boys, ages 5 to 19; students in public kindergartens and schools; those in public schools with innovative programs; and students from specialized schools for children and adults with language impairments. The adult sample of 36 women and 22 men ranged in age from 19 to 48 years; 38 had received higher education.

The psychologists administered the tasks individually or in small groups. Most had participated in a training program that included a seminar on the SDT.

## Results

Cognitive scores in Russia increased with age. This growth was considerable but uneven, with the greatest gains in the early school years, then beginning to slow at ages 12 to 13, with adults receiving the highest scores. A surprising finding in both Russia and the United States was that scores on the Drawing from Imagination and Drawing from Observation tasks were lower at ages 17 and 18 than at ages 15 to 16.

These investigators found the scores of Russian and American adults to be the same, but the scores of the Russian children and adolescents were often higher than scores of their American counterparts in predictive drawing, drawing from observation, and total test scores. On the other hand, American scores were higher on the Drawing from Imagination task. They attributed these findings to cultural differences, such as noting that manual skills are valued highly in Russia, where children usually are trained to use them early in their lives.

Investigators found no significant difference in the scores of children and adolescents with normal language skills and the scores of adolescents with language impairments, suggesting that the cognitive skills assessed by the SDT are independent of verbal skills.

They found no significant differences among children and adults from various regions of the Russian Federation, but they did observe differences between children attending regular public schools and those in schools with innovative programs.

Although the investigators found no differences between the sexes in cognitive content, considerable gender differences emerged in emotional content and in self-image. Females had higher, more positive scores in both categories.

In addition, they compared the frequencies of different responses. Although ambiguous, unemotional, and unclear drawings (3 points) predominated, investigators found strongly negative themes in emotional content three times more frequently among males (life-threatening relationships or sad or helpless solitary subjects, scoring 1 point).

At the same time, they found strongly positive themes three times more frequently among females (caring relationships or effective/happy solitary subjects, scoring 5 points) and moderately positive themes twice as frequently (friendly relationships or fortunate but passive solitary subjects, scoring 4 points).

Positive self-images also predominated among females, suggesting that females identified with powerful, beloved, or effective subjects (5 points) as well as with fortunate but passive subjects (4 points) three times more frequently than did males.

Similar gender differences in emotional content scores were found in the United States, as was reported in chapter 5. More than three times as many American males responded with strongly negative themes, scoring 1 point (17% males, 5% females), and more females than males responded with strongly positive themes, scoring 5 points (13% females, 9% males) and moderately positive themes (27% females, 15% males).

The reverse emerged in self-image scores. More American males than females scored 4 points (18% males, 12% females) and 5 points (18% males, 12% females), although neutral 3-point scores predominated (59% of males, 59% of females).

## The Draw a Story Assessment

Recently, three Russian clinicians administered the DAS task to groups of delinquent and nondelinquent children and adolescents in order to compare them with aggressive and nonaggressive groups of American adolescents (Kopytin, Svistovskaya, and Sventskaya, 2005). The 27 adolescents in the delinquent group had been diagnosed with social conduct disorder; they ranged in age from 10 to 14 years and included 6 girls and 21 boys. Many had been raised in residential institutions because they had been abandoned by or taken from their parents. All had demonstrated aggressiveness and several had attempted suicide. To develop a Russian control group, they also tested 25 children and adolescents without a diagnosis of social conduct disorder who also lived in an institution.

## Emotional Content

No significant cultural differences were detected in emotional content scores ($F$ [1,261] = .655; $p < .42$). This finding may reflect the dysfunctional family life experienced by respondents in both groups. The mean score of the American aggressive group was the lowest of all four groups. No child or adolescent in either group drew strongly positive fantasies scoring 5 points on either scale.

Similarities also appeared in the proportions of children and adolescents who drew strongly negative fantasies scoring 1 point in both emotional content and self-image, suggesting that they were depressed. In the Russian group, 19% of the aggressive adolescents and 4% of the controls scored 1 point on both scales; in the

American aggressive group, 17% of the aggressive group and 4% of the controls scored 1 point.

In addition, the control groups in both countries expressed more positive feelings than the aggressive groups, receiving higher scores in both emotional content and self-image.

## Self-Image

Highly significant cultural differences emerged in self-image scores. An analysis of variance (ANOVA) revealed a significant effect of nationality ($F$ [1,261] = 19.06; $p < .001$), the American students with higher scores than their Russian counterparts.

It was unexpected to find that the Russian groups not only had significantly lower self-image scores, but also that the scores of the delinquent Russian adolescents tended to be strongly negative, unlike their American counterparts, who tended to be strongly positive. The finding suggests that the Russian delinquent adolescents tended to be depressed as well as delinquent, unlike most of the American aggressive adolescents, although 5 of the 30 Americans also seemed depressed, scoring 1 point on both scales.

How can these differences be explained? Perhaps they are associated with the cultural differences that Bok (2003) described in her study of the nature of happiness. People in Latin American countries reported being happier on average than people in China, Japan, Korea, and countries recently under communist rule, who reported lower levels of satisfaction when responding to the question, "All things considered, how satisfied or dissatisfied are you with your life as a whole now?" Measured on a scale of 1 to 10, the mean score of the Russian respondents (4.2) was considerably lower than the mean score of the American respondents (7.4).

On the other hand, the disparity may reflect the difference between living at home with one's family and living in a psychiatric hospital, where the aggressive Russian adolescents were tested. Furthermore, they were not receiving psychotherapy—only psychotropic drugs. A previous study of American incarcerated, delinquent adolescents found that they, too, tended to draw sad rather than aggressive fantasies (Silver, 1996c).

## Comparing Aggressive and Nonaggressive Groups

As noted previously, an ANOVA found aggressiveness significantly related to scores on both scales; that is, the scores of the aggressive students were significantly lower in emotional content and significantly higher in self-image. In addition, a chi-square analysis revealed that aggressive students were significantly more likely than nonaggressive students to score 1 point in emotional content combined with 5 points in self-image, to a highly significant degree.

Although none of the American aggressive students drew fantasies with strongly positive emotional content (5 points), 4% of those in the control group drew strongly positive fantasies, such as caring or loving relationships, and five girls and one boy scored 5 points on both scales. Also in the control group, 12% drew moderately positive fantasies, such as friendly relationships or fortunate solitary subjects, compared with 7% of the aggressive students. On the other hand, more than three times as many aggressive American students (43%) drew strongly positive self-images, compared with 14% of the American control group, receiving significantly more positive self-image scores.

In self-image scores, no significant difference between the Russian delinquent and control groups emerged. In emotional content, however, the mean score of the Russian control group was significantly higher than the mean score of the delinquent group, in both self-image and emotional content. Unlike the American control group, only one in the Russian control group (0.04%) scored 5 points in emotional content, compared with 4% of the American controls. Additional findings were reported previously elsewhere (Silver, 2005).

The Russian investigators illustrated their findings with four response drawings, and for each drawing there was an American counterpart. For example, in both countries, an aggressive male adolescent selected stimulus drawings of the snake and the mouse (see figs. 12.1 and 12.2). Both drew the snakes devouring the mice, both stated that the mouse had entered the snake's territory, and both seemed to identify with their snakes, scoring 1 in emotional content and 5 in self-image. In the American control group, however, another youth who selected the snake and the mouse showed compassion, adding a drain pipe that enabled the mouse to escape (see fig. 12.3).

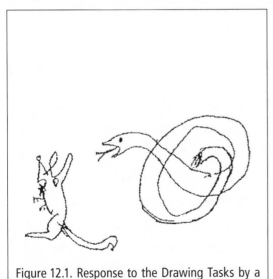

Figure 12.1. Response to the Drawing Tasks by a Russian Delinquent Youth.

Figure 12.2. Response to the Drawing Tasks by an American Aggressive Youth.

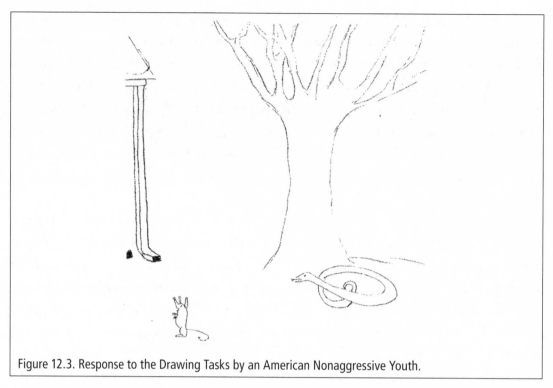

Figure 12.3. Response to the Drawing Tasks by an American Nonaggressive Youth.

The Russian investigators concluded that DAS provides a valid instrument for assessing the emotional needs and fantasies of delinquent adolescents. They found it helpful in understanding perceptions of self and others, establishing rapport with those who are unlikely to express their needs verbally, and providing interventions that reduce the risk of destructive or self-destructive behavior.

# Thailand

## The Silver Drawing Test

*Piyachat R. Finney*

Ms. Finney returned to Thailand after graduating from and teaching in the graduate program in expressive therapies at Lesley College in Boston. After serving as a clinician in the United States for seven years, Finney (1994) described her use of art therapy assessments. She used the SDT for access to the cognitive skills, creativity, and fantasies of her clients, and noted that newly admitted clients usually felt safe with the SDT. It reduced anxiety by enabling them to regulate distance and closeness, as well as maintain defenses in the first phase of a relationship. She found Burns and Kaufman's House-Tree-Person assessment useful in the middle phase of treatment, and both assessments useful as posttests.

After returning to Thailand, Finney taught university courses in art therapy to clinicians, social workers, counselors, and psychiatric nurses. Recently, she wrote that she finds the SDT an effective tool for evaluating levels of cognition as well as for evaluating impulsivity or attention/concentration. Parents were impressed that it helped her observe problem areas and strengths accurately.

In addition, she wrote:

> Since October 2001, in addition to using the SDT for an initial assessment in my private practice work with children, I have also used the *Drawing from Imagination Subtest* to evaluate the degree of aggressive behaviors in children who have been diagnosed as having Oppositional Defiant Disorder (ODD) and/or as having Depression (with depressive agitation). The pictures drawn by these youngsters often gave me a way to link the story content to their real life experiences. Moreover, the assessment shows an overview of not only their ability to process information, but also their level in receptive and expressive language areas. The written reports (with written consents from parents) were sent and shared with the children's treatment team members (psychiatrists in both public and private hospitals) and teachers at schools. This particular SDT assessment tool gives other professionals in the fields of Mental Health and Education another valuable perspective on the child's emotional states and his/her ability to communicate both verbally and nonverbally. (personal communication)

*Pornchit Dhanachitsiriphong*

One of Finney's students at Burapha University, Pornchit Dhanachitsiriphong, used the SDT as a pre- and posttest to assess the effects of an art program on male adolescents in a detention facility (1999). She selected her subjects from a group of 100 adolescents whose SDT cognitive scores were higher than the percentile rank of 75 and whose emotional content scores were lower than the percentile rank of 25. She then divided the sample into experimental and control groups, with six adolescents in each group.

The experimental group participated in art therapy and rational emotive therapy for 12 sessions during a period of three months, while the control group continued regular activities.

## Results

Following the experiment, Dhanachitsiriphong found the cognitive and emotional scores of the experimental group higher than control group scores to a degree significant at the .01 level of probability in the eight categories under consideration. The categories included scores obtained after the experiment in cognitive development, during a follow-up period in cognitive development, after the experiment in emotional development, after the follow-up period in emotional development, and other scores.

Dhanachitsiriphong observed that the SDT was useful for access to the unconscious, and translated the assessment into the Thai language for use in teaching as well as helping clients in nonprofit programs.

To illustrate, S, age 19, responded to the Drawing from Imagination task by choosing and simply copying stimulus drawings of a boy and an elderly man, but drew a man larger than a sad-looking boy. As he explained, his father had been ill and passed away while he was incarcerated. He longed to see his father, and wished some other delinquents would feel the same pain. Since his response ranked below the 25th percentile in emotional content and above the 75th percentile in cognitive content, it qualified S for the art program.

Responding again after the art program, S chose the boy, bed, and TV, drawing them in a room with pictures and a clock on the wall, and curtains billowing from an open window. As the art therapist explained, he was thinking about having his own bed and TV, adding that boys in the facility sleep on the floor in hot, poorly ventilated rooms.

The change in his drawings from bleak reality to hopeful fantasy, from 1 to 5 points in emotional content and self-image scores, suggests that it was caused by the intervention of 12 sessions in art therapy and rational emotive therapy over a period of three months.

The strongly negative responses of delinquent adolescents in Thailand seem no different from those of delinquent adolescents in the United State and Russia. To generalize, however, would require larger numbers, matched samples, and statistical analyses.

# Brazil

A group of art therapists and psychologists in Brazil standardized the SDT on approximately 2,000 children and adults (Allessandrini, Duarte, Dupas, & Bianco, 1998). They also examined responses for possible differences in schooling, gender, and type of school (public or private), and compared the performances of respondents in Brazil and in the United States. In translating the SDT manual into Portuguese, they made an adaptation to Brazilian culture in the Predictive Drawing task, substituting a soft drink for the ice cream soda, which is not widely consumed in Brazil. After administering the SDT and scoring responses, they developed norms and analyzed results.

The subjects included students in elementary and high schools, as well as three groups of adults: those whose education had been limited to elementary schools were placed in group 1; those who had attended high school in group 2; and those who had attended college in group 3.

The psychologists and art therapists tested 1,995 subjects in São Paulo. The largest city in Brazil, it receives heavy migration from elsewhere in the country and was considered representative of the Brazilian population. The children, ages 5 to 17, included subgroups based on grade, gender, and type of school; the adults, ages 18 to 40, were grouped on the basis of educational background. The testers selected at random 10 girls and 10 boys (or more) from at least three schools in each of 13 subgroups: one school in a central city area, another on the outskirts, and the third in between. Each subgroup of children and adults included at least 30 subjects.

The adult sample consisted of volunteers who were blue-collar workers and professionals in several companies and educational institutions. They included 196 women and 304 men, ranging in age from 18 to 40 years, with a mean age of 29 and a standard deviation of 8 years.

A team of psychologists and art therapists trained by the authors administered and scored the SDT. The investigators hypothesized that the SDT could measure manifestations of emotion, cognition, and level of development; that cognitive scores would improve with schooling; and that there would be significant emotional content in responses to the Drawing from Imagination task. They used an ANOVA to determine whether there were significant differences between groups.

## Results

The analyses yielded differences in school grade and type of school, increasing with age and grade level in subtest and total scores. The differences were significant at the .001 level of probability. Growth was more pronounced in the early grades. In general, the scores of private school students were higher than the scores of public school students. High school students were not differentiated either by grade or type of school. The mean scores of adults with limited education were below those of school-age children.

Their findings confirmed the dependence of cognitive scores on age and level of education, regardless of gender. No significant gender differences were found, although borderline differences emerged in the Predictive Drawing and Drawing from Observation tasks. No differences emerged among high school students either in grade or in type of school, but college graduates had higher mean scores than high school seniors. In both Brazil and the United States, the trend of growth in mean scores was similar, increasing gradually with grade and age level.

Among adults, analyses of variance confirmed the high correlation of SDT scores with level of education but not with gender. Among groups 2 and 3, who had from 7 to more than 11 years of schooling, nonsignificant gender differences emerged in predictive drawing, with superior performances among males. This finding was inconsistent with research findings in Australia, as will be discussed later in this chapter.

# The Silver Drawing Test and Draw a Story

Although the trend of mean scores was similar in both Brazilian and American cultures, the American scores were consistently higher in subtest mean scores and total scores, a finding that was inconsistent with the findings in Russia, as discussed previously.

No significant cultural differences were found in the emotional content of responses to the Drawing from Imagination task. In addition, the authors broke down the five SDT ratings of 1 to 5 points, ranging from strongly negative to strongly positive, classifying them into 21 specific items. For example, Brazilian items 1 to 5 included subjects who were sad, isolated, suicidal, dead, or in mortal danger. Items 11 to 13 included ambivalent content, unemotional content, and ambiguous or unclear content. They found more negative than positive ratings, and the rate of ambivalence was very high.

Similar emotional content was found in the responses of sixth-graders, twelfth-graders, and college students. They also shared a high level of ambivalence compared with the other groups. None of the Brazilian twelfth-graders responded with strongly negative content. Among seventh- and eighth-graders, however, strongly and moderately negative themes were frequent.

Nonemotional content predominated among Brazilian children from preschool to fourth grade. From fourth to sixth grades, the three neutral categories were more equally balanced, but in sixth grade, ambivalent content was more prevalent.

The Brazilian investigators found the rate of ambivalence consistently high. They interpreted this as demonstrating a tendency to see both sides of an issue, and concluded that the SDT offers an integrated form of evaluating subjects, especially those with learning disabilities, enabling clinicians to understand how they think and feel, and providing guidelines for treatment.

In our studies of students in the United States, the emotional content mean scores of male students, but not female students, paralleled the Brazilian finding of a tendency toward negative themes. On the other hand, the mean scores of our female students expressed ambiguous, unemotional, and ambivalent themes, paralleling the high rates of ambivalence found among Brazilian respondents of both genders.

To examine interscorer and test-retest reliability, three judges, working independently, scored responses by 32 children selected at random in all grade levels. Results indicated strong interscorer reliability, with correlation coefficients of .94, .95, and .95 in total SDT scores. To examine retest reliability, the SDT was administered twice to a group of 44 subjects after intervals of 15 to 30 days. Correlation coefficients ranged from .62 to .87, showing reliability.

# Use of the Silver Drawing Test and Draw a Story by Practitioners Abroad

## Australia

Glenda Hunter, a graduate student in the masters of education program at the University of New England in Armidale, New South Wales, used the SDT as well as four other assessments to examine individual and gender differences in Australia (Hunter, 1992).

Her subjects included 65 male and 128 female students, ages 15 to 53. Most of the males were enrolled in the university's engineering and construction apprenticeship courses; the female students, in office education courses.

Hunter used the mean ratings of two scorers to assess 11 variables based on the three SDT subtests: ability to sequence and predict horizontality and verticality (Predictive Drawing); ability to represent spatial relationships in horizontality, verticality, and depth (Drawing from Observation); and ability to select, combine, and represent, emotional expression, and language abilities based on the titles of responses (Drawing from Imagination). Hunter also grouped the variables into three components. Component 1 reflected originality in solving problems that were satisfying to the test taker rather than providing a correct solution to a problem. She defined these responses as *unrestricted* spatial thinking or problem solving, which included ability to select, to combine, and to represent.

Component 2 reflected *restricted* spatial thinking—that is, correct solutions to problems of representing spatial relationships in three dimensions and in sequencing. Component 3, which accounted for 11.1% of the variance (eigenvalue = 1.2), reflected ability to conserve and predict by visualizing changes in position while the properties of objects remain the same.

## Results

Two multivariate analyses of variance found significant gender differences in restricted and unrestricted spatial thinking or problem solving. The women had higher mean scores in unrestricted spatial thinking, performing better than the male students in the Drawing from Imagination task. The women also were superior on restricted tasks, which required defining visual-spatial relationships of objects in height, width, and depth and, to some extent, sequential order.

The contrast of gender was significant ($F$ [1,150] = 5.8; $p$ < .001). The associated univariate $F$ test for drawing from imagination was significant ($F$ [1,150] = 13.3; $p$ < .001, Eta2 = .08). In addition, the associated univariate $F$ test for drawing from observation was significant ($F$ [1,150] = 7.7; $p$ < .006, Eta2 = .05).

Drawing from imagination accounted for 33.3% of the variance (eigenvalue + 3.7) defined by the variables loading .81 or above (ability to select, combine, represent, and language). The variable projection (emotional content), which loaded .53, was not found significant. Predicting horizontality loaded .73 and predicting verticality loaded .71. Drawing from observation accounted for 17.6% of the variance with loadings of .78 or higher (height, width, and depth).

Hunter observed that the findings were consistent with the theory that cognitive skills evident in verbal conventions can be evident also in visual conventions. She also observed that the gender differences found in her study were worthy of consideration in developing course methodologies that may facilitate more effective learning outcomes for these college students.

## Turkey

Dr. Cagla Gur of Gazi University in Ankara, Turkey, used the SDT to determine the effectiveness of an experimental program for gifted six-year-old children, and to compare experimental and control groups, during the 2004–2005 school year (Gur, 2006). Children who demonstrated intelligence of 110 or higher on the Goodenough-Harris Draw-a-Man Test, and above 130 on the TKT 5–7 Test were selected for the experimental group, which included 26 girls and 26 boys. They attended 18 30-minute experimental art classes, three days a week for six weeks. The control group included children who received lower scores and did not participate in the program.

The first seven sessions of Gur's program were based on the developmental procedures used in the National Institute of Education Project (Silver et al., 1980), which used studio art experiences to develop the three independent concepts said to be fundamental in mathematics and reading: concepts of class inclusion and sequential order had been developed through the Drawing from Imagination task, and concepts of space, through the Drawing from Observation task, as was discussed in chapter 6. The next eleven sessions were developed by Gur.

Gur found that the children who participated in the experimental program showed improvement in each of the three cognitive skills to a degree that was significant at the $p < .001$ level of significance whereas no significant differences were found in the duration of preschool education ($p > .05$), or between genders ($p > .05$).

In addition, Gur found significant correlations between the SDT and the Goodenough-Harris Draw-a-Man Test ($n = 150$, $r = .49$; $p < .001$) as well as test-retest correlations ($n = 30$, SDT total 0.90; predictive drawing: 0.95; drawing from observation: 0.72; drawing from imagination: 0.96). The art procedures and tools used in the National Institute of Education Project are presented in chapter 13.

## Conclusion

The studies reviewed in this chapter suggest that the SDT is relatively free from cultural bias that favors some and discriminates against others. I am aware of only one cultural adaptation in administering the test: Allessandrini at al. changed the ice cream soda of the Predictive Drawing task into a plain soda to accord with Brazilian culture.

# Section IV

# Developmental Techniques and Concluding Observations

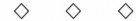

# Chapter 13

# Developmental Techniques

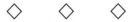

**B**efore reviewing the art techniques used to develop cognitive skill, this chapter discusses their underlying objectives.

## Objectives

### Developing Concepts of Space, Sequential Order, and Class Inclusion

The three concepts cited by Piaget (1970) as fundamental not only in mathematics and reading but also in all branches of knowledge seem no less fundamental in the visual arts. For example, the ability to form groups on the basis of class inclusion calls for the ability to select, combine, and represent. The painter selects and combines colors, and if the painting is representational, selects and combines images as well. The art techniques used to develop these concepts include drawing, painting, and modeling clay.

### Inviting Exploratory Learning

We can encourage children, adolescents, and adults to experiment with art tools and materials, protect them from interruptions, provide time for quiet reflection, and demonstrate suggestions on scrap paper. The time to intervene is when frustration seems imminent, such as someone struggling with a brush that is too large, too small, too wet, or too dry. We can invite exploratory learning by establishing an atmosphere in which independence and initiative are self-rewarding. Studio art experiences are often so rewarding that they are considered play instead of learning.

### Expanding the Range of Communication

We can provide a nonverbal channel through which to convey thoughts and feelings, encourage meaningful drawings rather than abstract designs, and emphasize content rather than form. We can also present tasks with many possible solutions rather than a single "correct" answer known in advance, and we can encourage diversity. Some individuals use poster paints instinctively in thin washes as though they were watercolors while others use them thickly, as though they were oils. Some prefer broad brushes; others, fine points. We can respect and encourage these differences.

### Building Self-Confidence

Responses to the Drawing from Imagination task tend to reveal how respondents feel about themselves and others. Shoemaker (1977) continues to investigate the special significance of the first drawing, and her observations are supported by first responses to the drawing task. Consider the self-image in figure 13.1, "Lyin' in the Livingroom," the first and only response by a young woman participating in a control group. Her drawing suggests self-confidence. On the other hand, consider figure 13.2, "Why Do You Bother Me?," the first response by Mike at age 8, and figure 13.3, "The Man in the Gabich Can," Mike's response at age 11. They seem to suggest that the worm, pig, and man in the garbage can represent himself, and reflect feelings of rejection and low self-esteem.

Studio art experiences provide opportunities for building self-confidence as well as tearing it down. Unlike a daydream, a fantasy on paper is vulnerable to anyone who feels qualified to judge. Building self-confidence does not call for insincere praise. Appreciating the subjective qualities of a drawing is valuing the person who drew it, and studio art experiences provide opportunities to elicit and develop the qualities that make each child, adolescent, or adult unique.

## Techniques for Developing Cognitive Skills

### The Ability to Select, Combine, and Represent through Drawings from Imagination

The ability to form groups on the basis of class or function involves making appropriate selections, associating them with past experiences, and combining them into a context, such as selecting words and combining them into sentences. Receptive language disorders are disturbances in the ability to make selections, and expressive

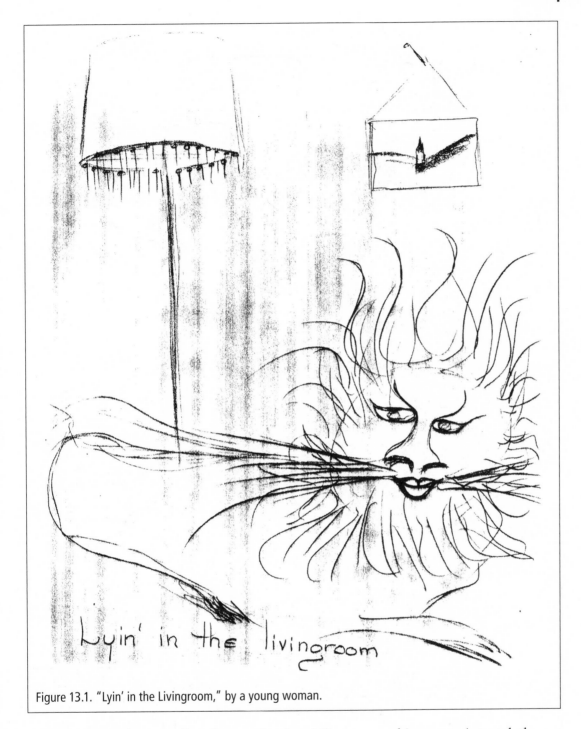

Figure 13.1. "Lyin' in the Livingroom," by a young woman.

language disorders are disturbances in the ability to combine parts into wholes, as was discussed in chapter 6.

As children develop they form groups based on perceptible attributes, such as colors or shapes. They progress to grouping based on function, such as showing what the subjects they selected do, and eventually acquire the abstract concept of a class or category.

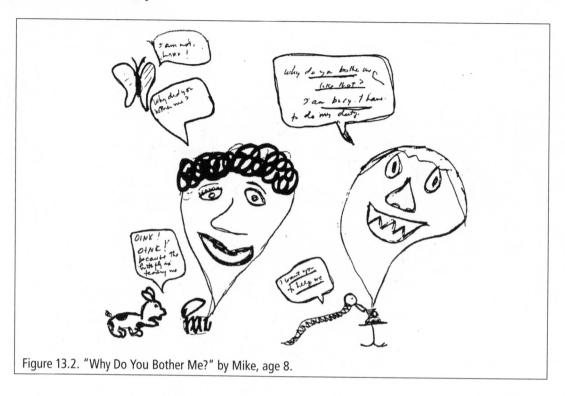

Figure 13.2. "Why Do You Bother Me?" by Mike, age 8.

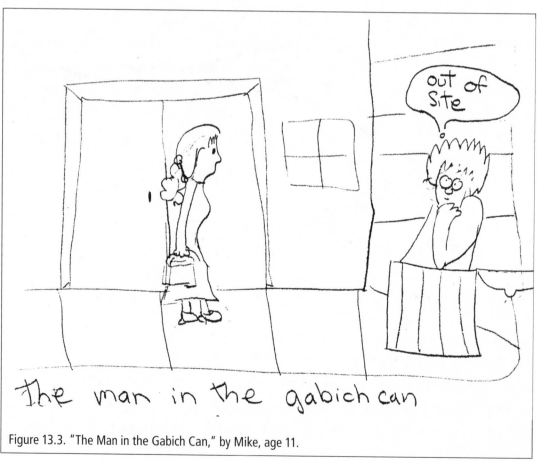

Figure 13.3. "The Man in the Gabich Can," by Mike, age 11.

Selecting and combining are also fundamental in creative thinking. The creative person tends to make unusual associations and then combine and represent them in innovative ways.

Studio techniques were attempts to develop these abilities by asking students to select stimulus drawings, combine the subjects selected, and represent them through images as well as words. The 50 stimulus drawings that were used to develop these abilities may be found in appendix C.

## Developing Concepts of Space through Drawing from Observation

In advance, I prepared an arrangement that included an orange and a cylinder made by rolling and taping a sheet of construction paper and arranging them on a table below eye level on another sheet of paper so that it appeared as a plane rather than a line, then placed the arrangement in the center of the room, surrounded by desks and chairs. After demonstrating with a quick sketch of the arrangement, I asked students to draw the arrangement from their individual points of view.

Instead of pointing out mistakes, I called attention to spatial relationships and provided time to draw the arrangement without interruptions or distractions to encourage exploratory learning.

## Developing Ability to Sequence through Painting and Modeling Clay

The concept of sequential order is said to be fundamental in reading and mathematics, as was discussed in chapter 6. It is no less fundamental in painting and sculpture, as in mixing colors and adding and removing lumps of clay.

The procedures for developing ability to sequence are described below in the 12-session art program that was used in the National Institute of Education Project reviewed in chapter 6.

# A 12-Session Art Program

The program presented here includes objectives and procedures for the first 12 sessions. Subsequent sessions should be based on the review of each student's strengths and weaknesses, and adapted to individual needs.

If the Silver Drawing Test is used before and after the program to note changes in ability, a minimum of 12 sessions (40 to 60 minutes each) should be planned. Preferably, for disabled students, the program should continue throughout the school year.

In addition to the specific objectives and procedures presented on the following pages, there are six general objectives and procedures that are appropriate to all the sessions.

# The Silver Drawing Test and Draw a Story

## Overview

| Objectives | Procedures |
|---|---|
| 1. To Develop Cognitive Skills | |
|    a. Focus attention | Set limits on activities, materials, and talk, emphasize demonstrations; avoid distractions; minimize talk while work is in progress. Then discuss and display work during the last 10 or 15 minutes of the session. |
|    b. Invite exploratory learning | Emphasize open-ended tasks (without single, "correct" solutions known in advance). |
|    c. Reinforce learning | Include kinetic as well as visual stimuli; provide time for quiet reflection; follow with verbal stimuli, introducing new words and encouraging the students to talk about their work. |
| 2. To Expand Communication by Developing Art Skills | Drawing, painting, and modeling clay. |
| 3. To Develop Creative Skills | Emphasize individuality and originality. |
| 4. To Build Self-Confidence | Emphasize reassurance and mutual respect; avoid situations that cause embarrassment, frustration, or anxiety; never work on a student's paper or sculpture—offer suggestions instead. |
| 5. To Set the Stage for Transfer | Try to make the learning experience so rewarding that students will use what they learn for their own purposes in their own ways in other situations. |
| 6. To Assess Ability and Record Changes | Keep a log of observations; score, photograph, or copy key works; date, number, and ask students to sign their work, leaving it with you until the end of the program. |

## First Session: Drawing from Imagination

*Materials:*

    stimulus drawing cards ( see appendix C group A, people and group C, things)

    paper: 8½ × 11″

    pencils with erasers

| Objectives | Procedures |
|---|---|
| 1. To develop ability to associate and form groups on the basis of class or function | |
|    a. Focus attention on associations | Cut the cards apart and present them in two adjacent groups, the word cards surrounded by the appropriate drawings. Demonstrate the task by selecting the SD prince from one group and the SD ladder from the other, then quickly sketch the prince climbing the ladder to rescue a child from a burning house. |

| Objectives | Procedures |
|---|---|
| b. Elicit associative thinking | Ask students to select one card from each group and draw a narrative picture: "Make your drawing tell a story about the picture ideas you choose. Show what is happening. Don't just copy these drawings; change them or create your own. Draw other things, too, to make your story more interesting." |
| c. Reinforce thinking | During the last 10 to 15 minutes, hold up the drawings one at a time. Encourage students to talk about their work, suggest a title, and write the titles along the bottom edges of the drawings. Ask students to return the cards to the groups where they belong when finished with them. |
| 2. Developing expressiveness | Emphasize the content of the drawing, their meanings rather than design or skill. |
| 3–6 | See overview. Make copies of first drawings to compare with later work. |

## Second Session: Drawing from Imagination

*Materials*

stimulus drawing cards groups B, animals, and D, places

paper: 8½ × 11″, 9 × 12″, and/or 12 × 18″

pencils with erasers

felt-tipped markers with both thick and thin points, in various colors

| Objectives | Procedures |
|---|---|
| 1. To develop ability to associate and form groups on the basis of class or function | |
| a. Focus attention | Present the stimulus drawing cards in two adjacent groups of animals and places, the word cards surrounded by the appropriate drawings. |
| b. Elicit associative thinking | Ask students to select two cards from different groups and again draw narrative pictures using small or large sheets of paper as they wish. Also offer choices among the marker colors. |
| c. Reinforce thinking | After drawings are finished, hold them up for discussion, including titles. Mix the cards and ask students to sort them by category. |
| 2. Develop expressiveness | Emphasize content rather than form. |
| 3–6 | See overview. |

# The Silver Drawing Test and Draw a Story

## Third Session: Painting

*Materials*

blue, red, and white poster paints, preferably in squeeze-jar containers (or paper cups)

paper: 12 × 18″

palette knives (or flat wooden sticks)

paper towels and sponges for cleaning up

newspapers for covering tables

smocks

| Objectives | Procedures |
|---|---|
| 1. To develop ability to sequence | |
| a. Focus attention on sequencing | Demonstrate mixing a series of blue tints by placing a dab of white on the upper right corner of a sheet of paper, and dab of blue on the upper left. With a palette knife or stick, mix a series of tints between them from left to right by adding more and more white to tints of blue. |
| b. Elicit associative thinking | Place dabs of blue and white on the upper left and right corners of students' papers and ask them to see how many tints of blue they can mix between the two colors. |
| c. Reinforce thinking | Encourage students to continue mixing or painting pictures on the rest of their paper: add more blue or white paint as needed on original dabs. As the paintings are finished, place them on the floor to dry, away from the painting area, and offer new sheets of paper. Limit second paintings to dabs of red on the upper left corner and white on the upper right corner, asking students to see how many tints of pink they can mix between them. They can then paint as they wish on the rest of their paper. |
| 2. Developing skill in painting and sensitivity to nuances of color | Emphasize form rather than content and the colors, shapes, and designs rather than narrative meaning. |
| 3–6 | See overview. |

## Fourth Session: Painting

*Materials*

yellow, blue, red, and white poster paints

paper: 12 × 18″ and 18 × 24″

1″ and pointed brushes

palette knives (or flat wooden sticks)

paper towels and sponges for cleaning up

newspapers for covering tables

smocks

| Objectives | Procedures |
|---|---|
| 1. To develop ability to sequence | |
| a. Focusing attention on sequencing | Place a dab of yellow on the upper right corner of each student's paper (12 x 18"), a dab of red on the upper left corner, and dab of blue on the lower right corner. |
| b. Elicit associative thinking | Ask students what they think will happen if they mix a series of color between the dabs. Have them test their predictions by mixing the colors. |
| c. Reinforce thinking | Encourage students to continue mixing and discovering colors, adding white to the lower left corner, replenishing colors as needed, and offering more paper for new paintings, either representational or abstract. |
| 2. To develop sensitivity and skill | Emphasize both form and content. |
| 3–6 | See overview. |

## Fifth and Sixth Sessions: Painting from Imagination

*Materials*

stimulus cards, Group D (places)

poster paints

paper: 12 × 18″ and 18 × 24″

1″ square and pointed brushes

palette knives (or flat wooden sticks)

paper towels and sponges for cleaning up

newspapers for covering tables

smocks

| Objectives | Procedures |
|---|---|
| 1. To develop ability to form concepts of space, order, and class | |
| a. Focus attention | Hold up one card at a time and ask, "Have you ever been to the beach? A farm? A volcano?" and so forth. |
| b. Elicit associative thinking | Ask students to paint pictures about a visit to some interesting place. "Show something happening there, and be sure to include yourself." |
| c. Reinforce thinking | In the time for discussion and display, point out horizontals, verticals, foregrounds, and backgrounds. Encourage each student to talk about his or her painting and give it a title. |
| 2. To develop art skills | Emphasize both form and content. |
| 3–6 | See overview. |

# The Silver Drawing Test and Draw a Story

## Seventh Session: Predictive Drawing and Painting

*Materials*

    toy boats (made from the cork of a bottle with the mast being a toothpick, and the keel a lump of clay) placed inside transparent jars filled with enough tinted water to float the boats

    toy fishing lines (strings weighted with lumps of clay and suspended from sticks); there should be one boat, jar, and plumb line for each four students

    8½ × 11″ paper

    pencils with erasers

    other art materials of choice

    a stool, chair, or pile of books so that boats can be presented at eye level on a horizontal surface

| Objectives | Procedures |
| --- | --- |
| 1. To develop concepts of horizontality and verticality | |
| a. Focus attention on horizontality | Put the boat in the jar; half fill with water and seal. Present the jar on its side at eye level on the table and ask, "How do you think the boat and the water would look if we tilted the jar up at one end? Would they still look the same or would they look different?" |
| b. Elicit associative thinking | Ask students to make a quick sketch. |
| c. Focus attention on verticality | Present the fishing line against a door or other vertical object so that the parallel between them is visible. Ask, "How do you think the fishing line would look if we move the pole up and down? Would it still look the same?" |
| d. Elicit associative thinking | Ask students to turn over their papers and make a quick sketch of the fishing pole and line. Invite students to test their predictions by manipulating the jars and lines. Be sure that the parallels (between table and water surface, door and plumb line) remain visible. |
| e. Reinforce thinking | Ask students to draw or paint a picture of someone fishing on a lake. In the discussion and display, encourage comments from each student, use the words horizontal, vertical, and parallel. |

## Eighth Session: Modeling Clay (Coils and Sonstroem Technique*)

*Materials*

> earth clay (or plasticene); in advance, prepare a fist-sized lump of clay for each
>    student and for yourself
>
> modeling tools (or pencils, paper clips)
>
> 18 × 24″ oilcloth (or newspaper or cardboard)
>
> wire for cutting clay into lumps
>
> plastic bags for storing sculptures

| Objectives | Procedures |
|---|---|
| 1. To develop concepts of space and ability to conserve | |
| a. Focus attention | Give each student a lump of clay and ask him or her to hold it in both hands. With eyes closed, ask them to twist, stretch, and hollow the clay, then examine the shapes that were formed. Demonstrate rolling clay into "snakes" and balls. |
| b. Elicit associative thinking | Ask students to divide their lumps of clay into two balls, and to make their balls the same by pinching clay from one and adding to the other. When they feel that the balls are the same, ask them to roll one into a snake, and ask if the ball and snake still have the same amounts of clay or if there is more in one than the other. Do not reveal correct answers. |
| c. Reinforce (or reconsider) responses | Ask students to change their snakes back into balls, and with their eyes closed and with one ball in each hand, again compare their weights. Say, "If they are not the same, make them the same, and roll one ball into a snake." Again, ask them to judge the amounts and explain. Leave the remaining time free for modeling from imagination. |
| 2. Developing art skills | Emphasize both form and content. |
| 3–6 | See overview. |

## Ninth Session: Modeling Clay (Slab Technique)

*Materials*

> earth clay (or plasticene); in advance, prepare a fist-sized lump of clay for each
>    student and for yourself
>
> modeling tools (or pencils, paper clips)
>
> 18 × 24″ oilcloth (or newspaper or cardboard)
>
> wire for cutting clay into lumps
>
> plastic bags for storing sculptures
>
> two flat sticks (about 12 × 1 × ¼″) and a wooden roller (about 12″) for each student
>    and yourself; these tools can be cut from old window shades

---

★ This conservation technique, described in 1b, was devised by Sonstroem (1966).

| Objectives | Procedures |
|---|---|
| 1. To develop concepts of space and ability to conserve | |
| a. Focus attention | Demonstrate how to form slabs by placing lumps of clay between parallel sticks and rolling them flat with both ends of the roller resting on the sticks. Slice off uneven edges, pressing them back onto the slab as needed and rolling again until the slab becomes a rectangle. Cut the rectangle into smaller rectangles and press pieces together, beginning to form a box. Demonstrate as quickly as possible, just long enough to convey the essential technique. |
| b. Elicit associative thinking | Ask students to roll out slabs and put them together into three-dimensional forms such as boxes, banks, or houses. |
| c. Reinforce thinking | Demonstrate, as needed, how to incise designs into slabs or add to the surface. Display and discuss finished work. |
| 2. To develop art skills | Emphasize both form and content. |
| 3–6 | See overview. |

## Tenth Session: Modeling Clay (Brick Technique)

*Materials*

> earth clay (or plasticene); in advance, prepare a fist-sized lump of clay for each student and for yourself
>
> modeling tools (or pencils, paper clips)
>
> 18 × 24″ oilcloth (or newspaper or cardboard)
>
> wire for cutting clay into lumps
>
> plastic bags for storing sculptures
>
> two flat sticks (about 12 × 1 × ¼″) and a wooden roller (about 12″) for each student and yourself; these tools can be cut from old window shades

| Objectives | Procedures |
|---|---|
| 1. To develop concepts of space, order, and class | |
| a. Focus attention | Demonstrate building "bricks" by forming clay into small blocks and pressing them together. Use this process to start to build a human form, beginning with feet, legs, and torso. Keep the demonstration brief. |
| b. Elicit associative thinking | Ask students to build human, animal, or other forms through this method. |
| c. Reinforce thinking | Ask students if they can put some of their sculptures together so that they convey meanings. Display, title, and discuss the works, as in previous sessions. |
| 2. To develop art skills | Emphasize both form and content. |
| 3–6 | See overview. |

## Eleventh Session: Drawing from Observation and Imagination

*Materials*

an orange

a cylinder (made by rolling and taping a sheet of blue construction paper); there
should be one orange and one cylinder for each four students

paper: 8½ × 11″

other art materials of choice

| Objectives | Procedures |
|---|---|
| 1. To develop awareness of spatial relationships (left/right, above/below, and front/back) | |
| a. Focus attention | Place the objects on a sheet of paper either on a low table, surrounded by four desks and chairs, or in the center of a large table. Center the orange on one corner of the paper and the cylinder on the opposite corner. The arrangement should be below eye level so that the paper is seen as a plane rather than a line. Demonstrate drawing the arrangement from observation with a quick sketch (just long enough to convey the essential technique). |
| b. Elicit associative thinking | Ask students to sketch the arrangement, including the paper base. |
| c. Reinforce thinking | Ask students to change seats with a classmate on the opposite side of the arrangement and sketch it again. Call attention to the fact that the cylinder appears to the left of the orange from one point of view, and to the right from another. Also call attention to the fact that the orange is in the foreground from one point of view, and in the background from another point of view. |
| d. To keep the emphasis open ended | Limit the time spent drawing from observation to about ten minutes, then ask students to draw pictures about their families during the remainder of the session: "Show your house and the people who live there with you." |

# The Silver Drawing Test and Draw a Story

## Twelfth Session: Drawing from Observation and Imagination

*Materials*

one sculpture made by each student in a previous class

drawing materials of choice

| Objectives | Procedures |
|---|---|
| 1. To develop concepts of space, order, and class | |
| a. Focus attention | Ask the students to select one of their own sculptures to draw from observation. |
| b. Elicit associative thinking | Ask them to make quick sketches, then turn their sculptures around, and sketch again. |
| c. Reinforce thinking | Instead of pointing out mistakes, say, "Is this the way you want it to look?" If not, offer suggestions on scrap paper and leave final decisions to students. |
| d. To keep the emphasis open ended | Limit the time for this drawing. Be guided by individual interests. Follow with free-choice drawing. |
| 2–6 | See overview. |

# Chapter 14

# Discussion and Conclusions

◇   ◇   ◇

This volume has presented new studies and reviewed others that made use of the stimulus drawing assessments. The studies examined responses to stimulus drawing tasks by individuals and groups. The responses provided opportunities to identify children and adolescents at risk for aggression and/or depression, the effects of therapeutic or developmental programs, and opportunities to evaluate cognitive and creative strengths and weaknesses across age groups, genders, and cultures. They also suggest an affirmative answer to a question raised in chapter 1: whether stimulus and response drawings tend to activate mirror neurons.

## Aggression

One of the recent studies found significant correlations between aggressive behavior and scores on the Draw a Story (DAS) rating scales. The experimental group of 30 children and adolescents who had been aggressive had significantly lower scores on the Emotional Content Scale and significantly higher scores on the Self-image Scale than the control group of 181 students who had not been aggressive. Aggression was significantly related to 1 point in emotional content combined with 5 points in self-image ($p < .001$), suggesting that this combination can serve as a first step in identifying students at risk.

Two subgroups of aggression also emerged: predatory and reactive. They differed in motivation and intensity and seem to call for different kinds of intervention.

## Predatory Aggression

This subgroup included aggressive students who seemed to identify with the assailants in their fantasies and amused by their helpless or frightened victims. All were boys. Five attended a school that did not have any preventive or therapeutic programs. Four of the five responded to the drawing task on several occasions, choosing the same stimulus drawings, and drawing predatory fantasies consistently. Shaun, Gus, and Sam drew knives poised above their victims. Carl drew the head and shoulders of a man in a dinosaur's mouth. They also showed consistency in concealing identities—knives thrown by invisible assailants and victims disguised as chicks. In addition, their drawings suggested morbid humor. Before suggesting that a particular student may be at risk for predatory behavior, additional information is needed, but no background histories for these students were available.

In the control group, 6 of the 181 students drew fantasies that suggest predatory aggression, 3% compared with 17% in the aggressive group.

## Reactive Aggression

This subgroup included five boys in the aggressive group who responded to the drawing task with fantasies about victims reacting to aggression with violence. Like those in the predatory subgroup, they scored 1 point in emotional content together with 5 points in self-image, but they tended to draw heroes fighting assailants, suggesting that they were motivated by a need to defend against threat instead of benefiting themselves. In the control group, no students responded with a drawing that suggested reactive aggression.

None of the five girls with histories of aggressive behavior drew fantasies about predatory aggression, but two suggested reactive aggression. Carol, age 17, drew a large chick protecting a small mouse, scowling at a middle-sized cat, and saying, "Pick on someone your own size." Harriet, age 16, seemed to identify with a passive princess "stuck in a castle, but a parachuting cowboy with a knife in his holster is trying to save her [from a dinosaur]." In the lower left corner of her drawing, however, a dead snake dangles from the beak of a chick; and in the lower right corner, a small mouse chases a larger cat.

Lanette and Victoria seemed to portray themselves as victims, scoring 1 point in both emotional content and self-image. Lanette, age 12, drew a snake attacking the groin of an armless girl who cries, "Help me!" She may have experienced sexual abuse, as suggested by her responses to the drawing task on several occasions. Her history includes an eating disorder and auditory hallucinations.

Victoria, age 17, chose the parachutist and the knife but changed the parachute into a balloon with an empty basket that "was cut with a knife and into the sea and was never found." Like Lanette, she had a history of abuse. She had been suspended from school for stealing, and sometimes seemed manic. Sherrie, age 17, also chose the chick. She described it as a baby bird that falls out of a tree looking for its mother.

## The Use of Humor

Additional differences between aggressive and control groups, as well as the subgroups, emerged in the use of humor and its absence.

None of the responses that suggested reactive aggression were humorous. In the aggressive group, however, more than 10 times as many students (20%) drew humorous responses to the drawing task, compared with 1.6% of the control group, and their humor tended to be strongly negative (mean score, 1.6 points). Four aggressive students used humor that was both morbid and homicidal, scoring 1 point; and none used humor that was playful, resilient, or ambivalent. In the control group, the humorous responses tended to be positive; their mean score was 3.3 points on the 5-point Humor Scale. Two students in the control group used resilient humor (4 points) and one used playful humor (5 points).

These findings suggest that there is an association between predatory aggression and humor that is both lethal and morbid, scoring 1 point, and since no humor appeared in the responses that suggested reactive aggression, the use of strongly negative humor also may distinguish predatory from reactive aggression.

## Preventive and Developmental Art Programs

Since predatory and reactive aggression differ in intensity and motivation, a combination of preventive programs may be more effective than a single one, according to MacNeil (2002), who recommends preventive strategies that encourage all members of the school community to work collectively toward a safer environment rather than emphasize law enforcement. He also recommends eliminating standing by passively, students and teachers who observe bullying behavior without attempting to stop it. Zero tolerance of bullying and prevention programs that encourage active participation by teachers and administrators, as well as students, have been successful. Other ways of controlling aggression redirect it toward substitute objects, and for some students, athletic competition can be effective in discharging aggression and teaching responsible self-control.

Another way is to provide programs in visual and fine arts. Each of the students whose responses suggest reactive rather than predatory aggression had been participating in art therapy programs for emotionally disturbed students. Their histories were available, and many revealed abuse and the death of parents, as well as maladaptive behaviors. The positive changes that appeared in their drawings and behaviors, as reported in chapters 4 and 11, seem causally related to the clinical interventions they received from the art therapists.

## Depression

The recent study found that 5 of the 30 students (17%) in the aggressive group drew strongly negative fantasies scoring 1 point on both the Emotional Content and Self-Image Scales, suggesting that they were depressed as well as aggressive. They also found that 8 students in the presumably normal control group (4%) scored 1 point on both scales, suggesting that they too might be depressed.

Another recent study found links between depression and reactive aggression. In the aggressive group, 5 of the 30 students scored 1 point in both self-image and emotional content, 17% compared with 4% of the nonaggressive control group. Four of these five aggressive students had been diagnosed with major depression previously, and were participating in art therapy programs. Jimmy, age 14, drew "When Dinosaurs Rule America," in which a parachute descends on a toothy dinosaur and two volcanoes erupt. The figure dangling from the parachute says, "I'm going to die!" When Jimmy finished drawing, he dictated a story that ended, "The plane was shot down by the dinosaur's breath attack. He says he is going to die because the dinosaur is in the castle. He's calling for backup but it won't come for a year." Jimmy had been diagnosed with major depression and attention deficit/hyperactivity disorder (ADHD), for which he takes medicine daily. It is not known whether he experienced abuse.

Joseph, age 10, drew "The Mouse Was Killing People from Around the World," but his mouse is small and helpless, almost invisible in the lava and rocks flying from a volcano so large that it overflows the drawing page. Joseph lashes out when frustrated or sad, or else withdraws completely. Also diagnosed with ADHD, he lives in a chaotic household. His father died prior to the onset of his aggressive and defiant behavior.

Ralph, age 12, drew "The Volcano Is Blowing Up the Castle," with a huge rock flying toward a small figure on a castle roof. Apart from aggressive behavior, little is known about Ralph's history.

Lanette and Victoria were the other two aggressive students whose responses scored 1 point in both emotional content and self-image.

In the control group, no students were known to be depressed, but eight responded with suicidal fantasies. They seemed to identify with subjects they portrayed as helpless, hopeless, lonely, or in mortal danger, scoring 1 point in both emotional content and self-image. Unfortunately, we were unable to identify them for clinical follow-up because they had responded anonymously.

Similar fantasies appeared in the responses of the 13 students in both groups who scored 1 point on both scales. Twelve of the 13 drew fantasies about life-threatening situations and subjects who were sad, hopeless, or helpless; and 11 of the 13 chose the stimulus-drawing knife and/or the volcano.

Differences between aggressive and nonaggressive groups also appeared. Suicidal fantasies and sad solitary subjects appeared only in responses by students in the control group, perhaps because students in the aggressive group had been acting out.

## Gender Differences and Similarities

Gender was significantly related to aggressiveness as well as to emotional content and self-image scores (Silver, 2002). In the aggressive group, boys had significantly higher, more positive scores than girls in self-image; and girls had significantly higher, more positive scores in emotional content.

No girls expressed predatory aggression, but five girls in the aggressive group expressed reactive aggression, and two of the five scored 1 point in both self-image and emotional content, suggesting that they were also depressed.

In the control group, more than twice as many girls received positive scores in emotional content (42% girls, 20% boys). In addition, their mean score was higher, and five girls but no boys scored 5 points in both emotional content and self-image. Seven girls but no boys drew strongly positive self-images about happy solitary subjects or loving relationships, and 18% of their responses, compared with 1% of the responses by boys, were moderately positive, scoring 4 points.

The findings support observations made by some investigators but not others. They support the observation that female aggressiveness is associated with sexual abuse, conduct disorder, and depression, but fail to support the observation that male aggressiveness tends to be overt and direct, whereas female aggressiveness tends to be indirect and covert. *Both* genders tended to express aggression indirectly in responding to the drawing tasks, disguising their assailants by making them invisible, or representing them as dinosaurs, snakes, or volcanoes. They also disguised their victims as chicks, mice, and cats.

Two previous studies found no gender differences in cognitive skills. The first study examined the spatial abilities of adolescents (Silver, 1996a). The SDT Predictive Drawing and Drawing from Observation tasks were administered to 33 girls and 33 boys ages 12 to 15 attending public schools in Nebraska, New York, and Pennsylvania. Their mean scores were analyzed using a computation of *t*-test scores. No significant differences emerged. The mean score of the girls was higher in ability to represent depth, but the probability was not significant.

The second study added responses to the drawing tasks by adults, ages 18 to 50 (mean age 26), bringing the total number of respondents to 88 males and 88 females (Silver, 1998a). Again, no significant gender differences in their scores emerged. Both males and females received lower scores in verticality than horizontality. When responses were examined individually, however, a nine-year-old girl and a male art director received the highest scores in verticality, whereas two male psychologists received the lowest scores in verticality.

## Age Differences and Similarities

More senior women than any other age or gender group drew fantasies about assaultive relationships, as measured by the SDT responses of 531 subjects in five age groups ranging from children as young as seven to senior adults (Silver, 1993a, 1993b, 2002). The converse age and gender interaction was found for caring relationships. The proportion of younger men who drew fantasies about caring relationships exceeded the proportion of younger women, as well as the proportion of all other male age groups. Females showed a significantly higher frequency of caring relationships across age groups, while males showed age variability.

In drawing about relationships, more senior men drew fantasies about stressful relationships than any other age or gender group. Although negative attitudes predominated among senior adults, they used humor more often than did any other age group. Their humor tended to be self-disparaging, whereas the humor of adolescents tended to be disparaging, ridiculing others.

## Cognitive and Creative Strengths and Weaknesses

Section 2 of this volume reviewed why and how the SDT assessment was developed, its reliability, its validity, normative data, and reports from practitioners who used it to assess the cognitive skills of clinical and nonclinical populations. It also includes a 12-session program for developing cognitive skills (chapter 13), reports by practitioners who used both the SDT and DAS to assess students with special needs (chapter 11), and new findings about creativity, as measured by the SDT Drawing from Imagination task.

Some key findings are summarized below.

## Creativity

Kopytin and Svistovskaya (2005) found significant correlations between the scores of Russian students in Ability to Represent in the SDT Drawing from Imagination task (the ability for assessing creativity) and their scores in two tests that were designed to assess creativity, the Torrance Test of Creative Thinking (Torrance, 1984), and the Creativity Assessment Packet (Williams, 1980), as reported in chapter 12. These correlations provide additional support for previous findings about the creativity of American students.

## Comparing Students with and without Hearing Impairments

Originally, the SDT was designed to assess the cognitive skills of children with auditory and language impairments, as discussed in chapter 6. Subsequently the scores of students with and without hearing impairments were compared. The hearing-impaired group included 13 girls and 14 boys, ages 9 to 11, all fourth-graders in an urban nonresidential school for deaf students. The hearing group included 14 girls and 14 boys attending two public elementary schools, matched in age and selected at random.

It was unexpected to find that the deaf children had higher scores than the hearing children in vertical orientation, and that no significant differences emerged in Drawing from Observation or Predictive Drawing task scores. The hearing children had significantly higher scores in the Drawing from Imagination task, as might be expected.

Russian investigators found no significant differences between the SDT scores of children and adolescents with and without language impairments, and concluded that the cognitive skills assessed by the SDT are independent of verbal skills.

Another unexpected finding emerged when a few teachers and psychologists confused spatial relationships in responding to the Drawing from Observation and Predictive Drawing tasks, and more than a few drew houses perpendicular to the slope, or drew lines parallel to the sides of the tilted bottle (see chapter 8). These adults may have had subtle cognitive dysfunctions overlooked because our schools tend to emphasize verbal abilities and disregard spatial abilities.

# Using the SDT and DAS Together

Linda Jo Pfeiffer, chairperson of the Clinical Art Therapy Department of Miami–Dade County Public Schools, described the department's use of both assessments, and five art therapists described their work with students individually. They use DAS when a student's SDT scores 1 point in both emotional content and self-image, or

1 point in emotional content combined with 5 points in self-image, to determine whether the student has problems that need to be addressed immediately.

## Cultural Differences and Similarities

When investigators in Australia, Brazil, Russia, Thailand, and the United States examined responses to DAS and the SDT, they found cultural differences and similarities in emotional content, self-images, and cognitive scores.

Comparing the aggressive groups in America and Russia, significant cultural differences emerged in self-image scores. The Russian delinquent group had significantly lower, more negative self-images than the American aggressive group, which tended to have strongly positive self-images. Perhaps these scores are associated with cultural differences, or reflect the differences between living at home with one's family and living in a psychiatric hospital (where the Russian delinquent adolescents were tested).

On the other hand, cultural similarities emerged in the number of children and adolescents who scored 1 point in both emotional content and self-image. The mean score of the American aggressive group was the lowest of all four groups. Males had lower, more negative scores than females, and positive themes predominated among females. No respondent in either country drew a strongly positive fantasy scored 5 points, perhaps reflecting the abandonment and dysfunctional family life experiences by respondents in both countries.

In Thailand, the sad fantasies of incarcerated adolescents were like the sad fantasies of adolescents in the United States.

Comparing respondents in Brazil and the United States, no significant cultural differences emerged in the emotional content of responses to the SDT Drawing from Imagination task. The neutral 3-point score predominated in Brazil, and males tended to draw more negative fantasies than females, also found in the United States and Russia.

When responses by Hispanic and non-Hispanic students in the United States were compared, minor differences appeared in total emotional content scores; but when negative scores were examined separately, more than twice as many Hispanic students scored 1 point. The finding reversed in responses that scored 2 points. When positive scores were examined separately, fewer Hispanic students scored 4 points but more scored 5 points. The Hispanic group had more positive self-images; 40% scored 5 points on the Self-Image Scale, compared with 27% of the American students.

In cognitive scores, the trend of mean scores in the United States and Brazil was similar, but the Brazilian scores were consistently lower in total cognitive scores and subtest mean scores. The reverse appeared in some Russian and American SDT scores. As found by the Russian investigators, the American students had lower total scores as well as lower scores in the Predictive Drawing and Drawing from Observation tasks, but higher scores in the Drawing from Imagination task.

In all three countries, cognitive scores increased with age and level of education, adults receiving the highest scores.

No gender differences in cognitive skills were found in the studies by American and Russian investigators, but the Australian investigator found that women had higher scores than men in the Drawing from Imagination and Drawing from Observation tasks.

It may be that the similarities across cultures are biological and the differences cultural, such as deciding what children should learn, and how they should be taught. As Kopytin (2002) has observed, "manual skills" are valued highly in Russia, where children are trained to develop them early in life. In American schools, they seem valued less highly.

## Concluding Observations

The findings of the new studies, like previous findings, seem to support the premise that responses to these stimulus drawing tasks can bypass language deficiencies and provide access to thoughts and feelings that may be inaccessible through words. They also suggest that the experimental tasks heighten awareness, develop conceptual thinking, and provide opportunities to sense what respondents experience.

The findings were both quantitative and qualitative, and I believe we need both. For example, the differences between reactive and predatory aggression that appeared in responses by individuals and subgroups disappeared in groups large enough for statistical analysis. On the other hand, without statistical analyses, findings would be limited to subjective observations and conjecture.

The findings also suggest an affirmative answer to a question raised in the introduction—whether stimulus and response drawings tend to activate mirror neurons. In addition, the findings suggest that Draw a Story and the Silver Drawing Test could be useful not only to mental health professionals but also to educators, and particularly, art therapists and art educators whose own studio experiences would seem to enhance sensitivity to the fears, angers, desires, and intentions, expressed nonverbally through drawings.

# Section V

# Appendices

◇    ◇    ◇

# The Silver Drawing Test of Cognition and Emotion

◇    ◇    ◇

## Drawing What You Predict, What You See, and What You Imagine

*Rawley A. Silver, EdD, ATR-BC*

Name........................... Age............ Sex.............. Date....................
.................................................................................................

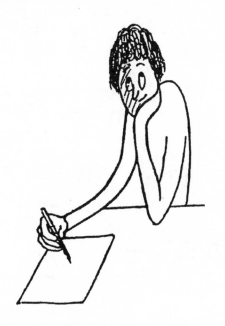

*© 1983–2007 by Rawley Silver. Reprinted with permission for personal use only.*

## Appendix A: The Silver Drawing Test of Cognition and Emotion

## The SDT Predictive Drawing Task

Suppose you took a few sips of a soda, then a few more, and more, until your glass was empty. Can you draw lines in the glasses to show how the soda would look if you gradually drank it all?

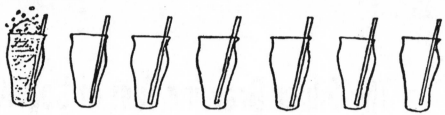

Suppose you tilted a bottle half filled with water. Can you draw lines in the bottles to show how the water would look?

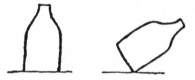

Suppose you put the house on the spot marked x. Can you draw the way it would look?

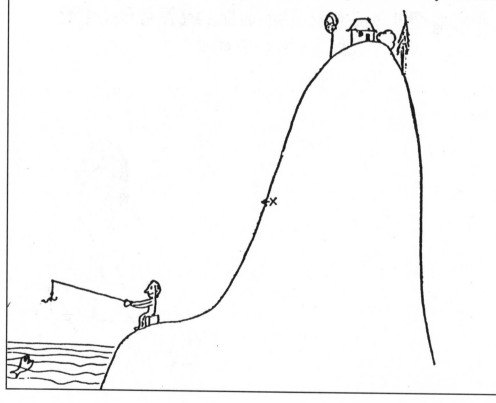

© 1983–2007 by Rawley Silver. Reprinted with permission for personal use only.

## The SDT Drawing from Observation Task

Have you ever tried to draw something just the way it looks? Here are some things to draw. Look at them carefully, then draw what you see in the space below.

© 1983–2007 by Rawley Silver. Reprinted with permission for personal use only.

## Appendix A: The Silver Drawing Test of Cognition and Emotion

# Drawing What You Imagine

### Form A, Silver Drawing Test

Choose two picture ideas and imagine a story — something happening between the pictures you choose.

When you are ready, draw a picture of what you imagine. Show what is happening in your drawing. You can make changes and draw other things too.

When you finish drawing, write a title or story. Tell what is happening and what may happen later on.

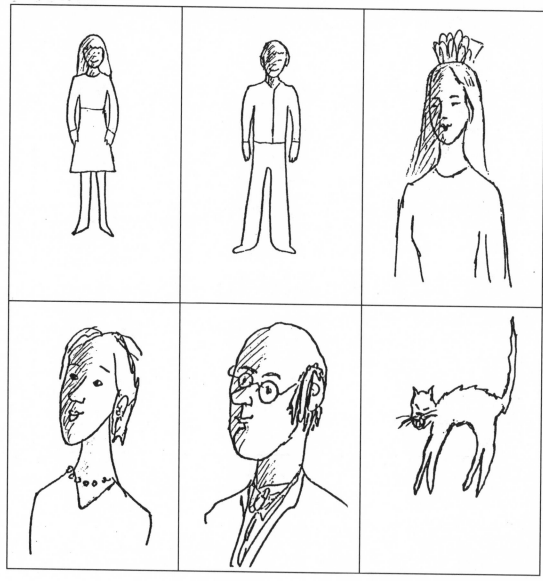

© 1983–2007 by Rawley Silver. Reprinted with permission for personal use only.

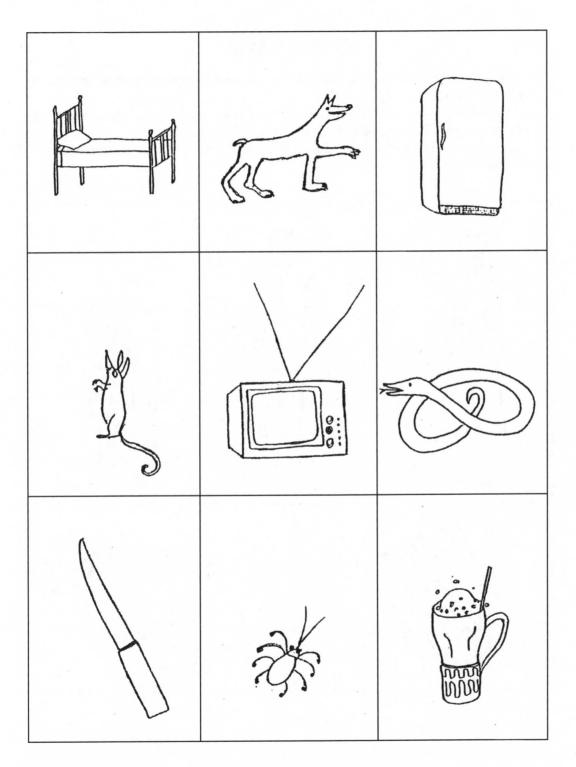

© 1983–2007 by Rawley Silver. Reprinted with permission for personal use only.

# Drawing What You Imagine

## Form B, Silver Drawing Test

Choose two picture ideas and imagine a story—something happening between the pictures you choose.

When you are ready, draw a picture of what you imagine. Show what is happening in your drawing. You can make changes and draw other things too.

When you finish drawing, write a title or story. Tell what is happening and what may happen later on.

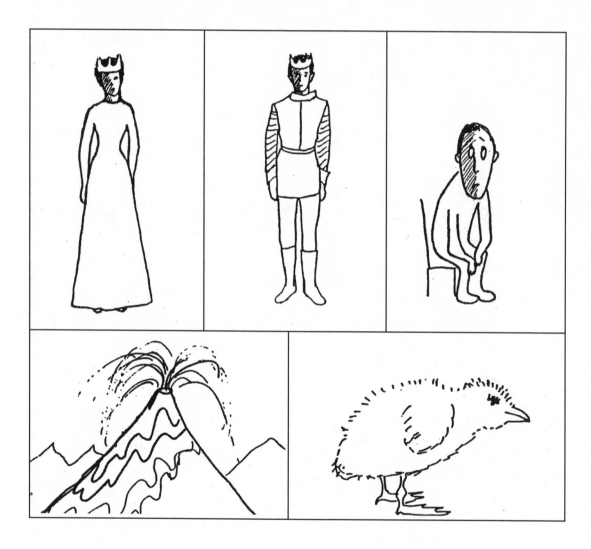

© 1983–2007 by Rawley Silver. Reprinted with permission for personal use only.

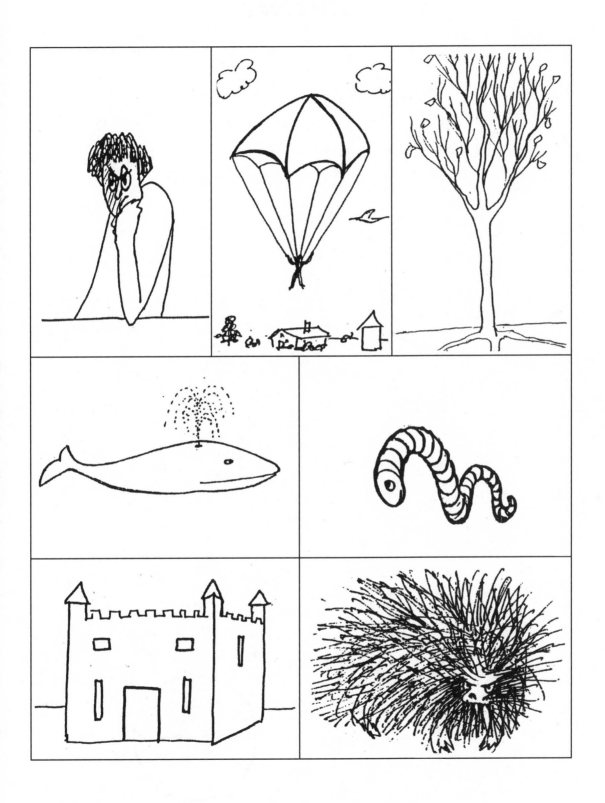

© 1983–2007 by Rawley Silver. Reprinted with permission for personal use only.

# SDT Layout Sheet

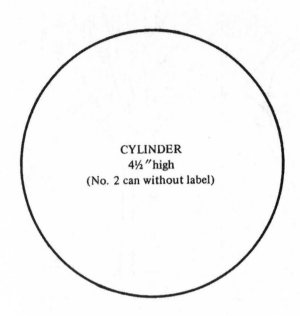

CYLINDER
4½″ high
(No. 2 can without label)

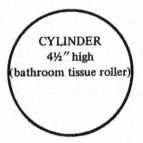

CYLINDER
4½″ high
(bathroom tissue roller)

© 1983–2007 by Rawley Silver. Reprinted with permission for personal use only.

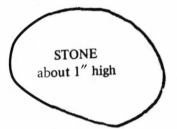

STONE
about 1″ high

CYLINDER
11″ high
(paper towel roller)

## Appendix A: The Silver Drawing Test of Cognition and Emotion

# The SDT Drawing from Imagination Task

**Drawing**

Story:_____

_____

_____

_____

_____

<u>Please fill in the blanks below:</u>

First name _____ Sex_____ Age _____ Location (state): _____Date:_____

Just now I'm feeling _____very happy _____O.K. _____angry _____frightened _____sad

© 1983–2007 by Rawley Silver. Reprinted with permission for personal use only.

## SDT Classroom Record Sheet

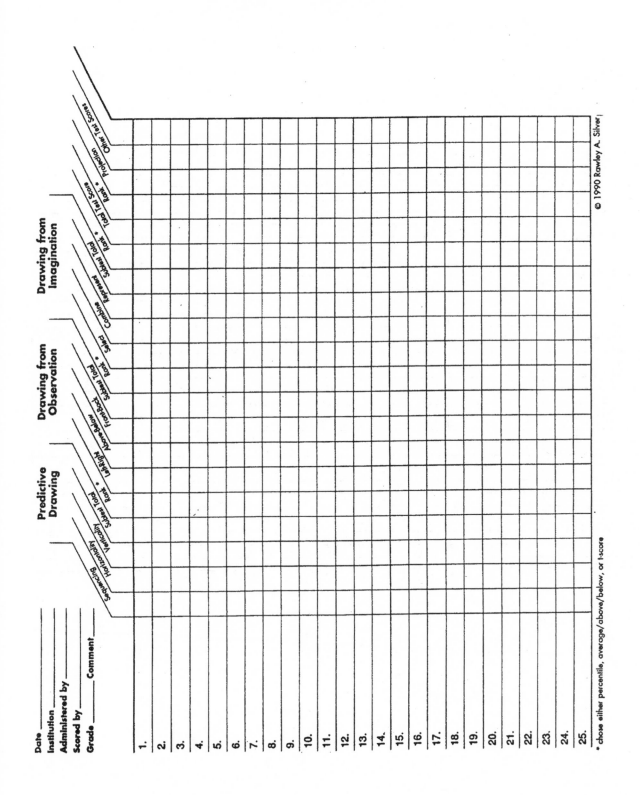

© 1990 Rawley A. Silver

\* chose either percentile, average/above/below, or t-score

# Appendix A: The Silver Drawing Test of Cognition and Emotion

## Record Sheet for Responses to the SDT Drawing from Imagination Task

Date _____
Administered by _____
Scored by _____
Institution _____

| First Name ID or Name | Age | EC | S-I | Humor | Title | Notes |
|---|---|---|---|---|---|---|
| 1. | | | | | | |
| 2. | | | | | | |
| 3. | | | | | | |
| 4. | | | | | | |
| 5. | | | | | | |
| 6. | | | | | | |
| 7. | | | | | | |
| 8. | | | | | | |
| 9. | | | | | | |
| 10. | | | | | | |
| 11. | | | | | | |
| 12. | | | | | | |
| 13. | | | | | | |
| 14. | | | | | | |
| 15. | | | | | | |
| 16. | | | | | | |
| 17. | | | | | | |
| 18. | | | | | | |
| 19. | | | | | | |
| 20. | | | | | | |
| 21. | | | | | | |
| 22. | | | | | | |
| 23. | | | | | | |
| 24. | | | | | | |
| 25. | | | | | | |
| 26. | | | | | | |
| 27. | | | | | | |
| 28. | | | | | | |
| 29. | | | | | | |
| 30. | | | | | | |

Copyright 1987 Rawley Silver

# Forms for Assessing Individual Responses to the Silver Drawing Test of Cognition and Emotion (SDT)

Name: _____ Age: _____Sex: _____ Date: _____

School: _____ Administered by: _____

The SDT is designed to assess cognitive development and to screen for emotional problems. The SDT includes three tasks: Predictive Drawing, to assess the ability to sequence and predict changes in the appearance of objects; Drawing from Imagination, to assess the emotional content of responses, as well as assess three cognitive skills; and Drawing from Observation, to assess concepts of space.

## The Predictive Drawing Task

*Guidelines for Scoring*

### Predicting a Sequence

| | |
|---|---|
| 0 points | No sequence representing the soda in the glasses |
| 1 point | Incomplete sequence |
| 2 points | Two or more sequences |
| 3 points | Descending series of lines with corrections (trial and error) |
| 4 points | A sequence with unevenly spaced increments but no corrections |
| 5 points | A sequence with evenly spaced increments and no corrections (systematic) |

*Note:* The sequence does not have to continue to the bottom of the glass

### Predicting Horizontality*

| | |
|---|---|
| 0 points | No line representing water surface is inside the tilted bottle |
| 1 point | Line parallels bottom or sides of tilted bottle (suggesting that the frame of reference is inside the bottle) |
| 2 points | Line almost parallels bottom or side of tilted bottle |
| 3 points | Line is oblique (suggesting that the frame of reference is external but not related to the table surface) |
| 4 points | Line seems related to the table surface but is not parallel |
| 5 points | Line is parallel to table surface within 5 degrees |

### Predicting Verticality*

| | |
|---|---|
| 0 points | No representation of the house or, if examinee is younger than five years, the house is inside the mountain |
| 1 point | House is approximately perpendicular to the slope. |
| 2 points | House is neither perpendicular nor vertical, but on a slant or upside down |
| 3 points | House is vertical but has inadequate support; may be entirely inside the mountain if examinee is older than five years |
| 4 points | House is vertical but has inadequate support, such as partly inside the mountain |
| 5 points | House is vertical, supported by posts, columns, platforms, or other structures |

*Note: The tasks for predicting horizontality and verticality are adapted from experiments by Piaget and Inhelder (1967).

© 1983–2007 by Rawley Silver. Reprinted with permission for personal use only.

# Appendix A: The Silver Drawing Test of Cognition and Emotion

## The Drawing from Observation Task

Sketches of the arrangement are shown below. The front view can serve as the criterion for drawings scored 5 points.

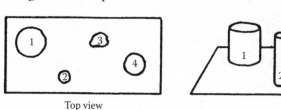

Top view  Front view

When scoring, note that cylinder #1 is the widest, #4 is the tallest, #2 is in the foreground, and the stone, #3, is behind and between #2 and #4.

To examinees seated toward the left, #2 appears farther from #1 and closer to #3.

To examinees seated toward the right, #2 appears farther from #3 and closer to #1.

*Guidelines for Scoring*

### Horizontal (Left/Right) Relationships

0 points  Horizontal relationships are confused; no objects are in the correct left-right order

1 point  Only one object is in the correct left-right order

2 points  Two objects are in the correct left-right order

3 points  Three adjacent objects or two pairs of objects are in the correct left-right order.

4 points  All four objects are approximately correct in order but not carefully observed or represented

5 points  All objects are in the correct left-right order

### Vertical (Above/Below) Relationships (Height)

0 points  All objects are flat; no representation of height

1 point  All objects are about the same height

2 points  Two objects (not necessarily adjacent) are approximately correct in height

3 points  Three objects (not necessarily adjacent) are approximately correct in height

4 points  All four objects are approximately correct in height but are not carefully observed and represented

5 points  All vertical relationships are represented accurately

### Front/Back Relationships (Depth)

0 points  All objects are in a horizontal row even though arrangement was presented below eye level, or no adjacent objects are correctly related in depth

1 point  One object is above or below a baseline (drawn or implied), or front-back relationships are incorrect

2 points  Two objects (not necessarily adjacent) are approximately correct in front-back relationships

3 points  Three adjacent objects or two pairs of objects are approximately correct in front-back relationships

4 points  All four objects are approximately correct in front-back relationships but not well observed and represented

5 points  All front-back relationships are represented accurately and the layout sheet is included in the drawing

© 1983–2007 by Rawley Silver. Reprinted with permission for personal use only.

# Appendix A: The Silver Drawing Test of Cognition and Emotion

## The Drawing from Imagination Task

*Scales for Assessing Cognitive Content*

### Ability to Select (Content or Meaning of the Response)

| | |
|---|---|
| 0 points | No evidence of selecting |
| 1 point | Perceptual level: single subject, or subjects unrelated in size or placement |
| 2 points | Subjects may be related in size or placement but there is no interaction |
| 3 points | Functional level: concrete, shows what subjects do, or what is done to them |
| 4 points | Descriptive rather than abstract or imaginative |
| 5 points | Conceptual level: imaginative, well-organized idea; implies more than is visible, or shows other ability to deal with abstract ideas |

### Ability to Combine (The Form of the Drawing)

| | |
|---|---|
| 0 points | Single subject, no spatial relationships |
| 1 point | Proximity: subjects float in space, related only by proximity |
| 2 points | Arrows, dotted lines, or other attempts to show relationships |
| 3 points | Baseline: subjects are related to one another along a baseline (real or implied) |
| 4 points | Beyond the baseline level, but much of the drawing area is blank |
| 5 points | Overall coordination; shows depth or takes into account the entire drawing area, or else includes a series of two or more drawings |

### Ability to Represent (Concepts and Creativity in the Form, Content, Title, or Story)

| | |
|---|---|
| 0 points | No evidence of representation |
| 1 point | Imitative: copies stimulus drawings or uses stick figures or stereotypes |
| 2 points | Beyond imitation, but drawing or ideas are commonplace |
| 3 points | Restructured: changes or elaborates on stimulus drawings or stereotypes |
| 4 points | Beyond restructuring: moderately original or expressive |
| 5 points | Transformational: highly original, expressive, playful, suggestive, or uses metaphors, puns, jokes, satire, or double meanings |

*© 1983–2007 by Rawley Silver. Reprinted with permission for personal use only.*

# Appendix A: The Silver Drawing Test of Cognition and Emotion

## Scale for Assessing Emotional Content

____1 point: strongly negative emotional content; for example:

Solitary subjects portrayed as sad, helpless, isolated, suicidal, dead, or in mortal danger

Relationships that are murderous or life threatening

____2 points: moderately negative emotional content; for example:

Solitary subjects portrayed as frightened, angry, dissatisfied, assaultive, or unfortunate

Relationships that are stressful, hostile, destructive, or unpleasant

____2.5 points: ambiguous or ambivalent emotional content suggesting unpleasant or unfortunate outcomes

____3 points: neutral emotional content; for example, ambivalent, both negative and positive; unemotional, neither negative nor positive; or ambiguous or unclear

____3.5 points: ambiguous or ambivalent emotional content suggesting hopeful, pleasant, or fortunate outcomes

____4 points: moderately positive emotional content; for example:

Solitary subjects portrayed as fortunate but passive, enjoying, or being rescued

Relationships that are friendly or positive

____5 points: strongly positive themes; for example:

Solitary subjects portrayed as effective, happy, or achieving goals

Relationships that are caring or loving

© 1983–2007 by Rawley Silver. Reprinted with permission for personal use only.

## Scale for Assessing Self-Image

____1 point: morbid fantasy; respondent seems to identify with a subject portrayed as sad, helpless, isolated, suicidal, dead, or in mortal danger

____2 points: unpleasant fantasy; respondent seems to identify with a subject portrayed as frightened, frustrated, or unfortunate

____2.5 points: unclear or ambivalent self-image with negative outcome; respondent seems to identify with a subject who appears unfortunate or likely to fail

____3 points: ambiguous or ambivalent fantasy; respondent seems to identify with a subject portrayed as ambivalent or unemotional, or else the self-image (such as the narrator) is unclear or invisible

____3.5 points: unclear, ambivalent, or negative self-image, but outcome seems positive; respondent seems to identify with a subject who appears likely to achieve goal

____4 points: pleasant fantasy; respondent seems to identify with a subject portrayed as fortunate but passive, such as being rescued

____5 points: wish-fulfilling fantasy; respondent seems to identify with a subject who is powerful, assaultive, loved, or achieving goals

© 1983–2007 by Rawley Silver. Reprinted with permission for personal use only.

## Scale for Assessing the Use of Humor

___1 point: lethal and morbid humor; for example:

Amused by subject(s) dying painfully or in mortal danger and overtly expressing pain and/or fear, either through words or images

___1.5 points: lethal but not morbid humor; for example:

Amused by subject(s) disappearing, dead, or in mortal danger but not expressing pain and/or fear, either through words or images

___2 points: disparaging humor; for example:

Amused by a principal subject who is unlike the respondent (such as of the opposite gender) and unattractive, frustrated, foolish, or unfortunate, but not in mortal danger

___2.5 points: self-disparaging humor; for example:

Uses personal pronoun and/or is amused by a principal subject who is like the respondent as well as unattractive, frustrated, foolish, or unfortunate, but not in mortal danger

___3 points: ambiguous or ambivalent humor (neutral); for example:

Meaning or outcome is both negative and positive, neither negative nor positive, or unclear

___4 points: resilient humor (more positive than negative); for example:

Principal subject(s) overcomes adversity or outcome is hopeful or favorable

___5 points: playful humor (entirely positive); for example:

Kindly, absurd, or with play on words, such as rhymes or puns

## Comments or Recommendations:

_____

_____

_____

_____

_____

_____

_____

_____

_____

© 1983–2007 by Rawley Silver. Reprinted with permission for personal use only.

## Appendix A: The Silver Drawing Test of Cognition and Emotion

# Silver Drawing Test Assessment

Name: _____ Age: _____ Sex: _____ Date: _____

School: _____ Administered by: _____

Subtest _____ Pretest _____ Norm _____

Score _____ Description _____ Score _____

Predictive Drawing

Drawing from Observation

Ability to Select

Ability to Combine

Creativity (Ability to Represent)

Emotional Content

Self-Image

Use of Humor

Subtest _____ Posttest_____ Norm_____

Score _____ Description _____ Score _____

Predictive Drawing

Drawing from Observation

Ability to Select

Ability to Combine

Creativity (Ability to Represent)

Emotional Content

Self-Image

Use of Humor

Behaviors, Relationships, and/or Recommendations

_____

_____

_____

*2002, 2006 Rawley Silver.*

# Draw a Story

◇    ◇    ◇

## Draw a Story

### Rawley Silver, EdD, ATR-BC

Name...........................................Age...........Sex..............Date...............

.........................................................................................................

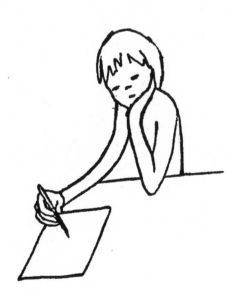

© 1983–2007 by Rawley Silver. Reprinted with permission for personal use only.

# Draw a Story

## Form A

Choose two of these drawings and imagine a story—something happening between the subjects you choose.

When you are ready, draw a picture of what you imagine. Make your drawing tell the story. Show what is happening. Feel free to change these drawings and to add your own ideas.

When you finish drawing, write the story in the place provided.

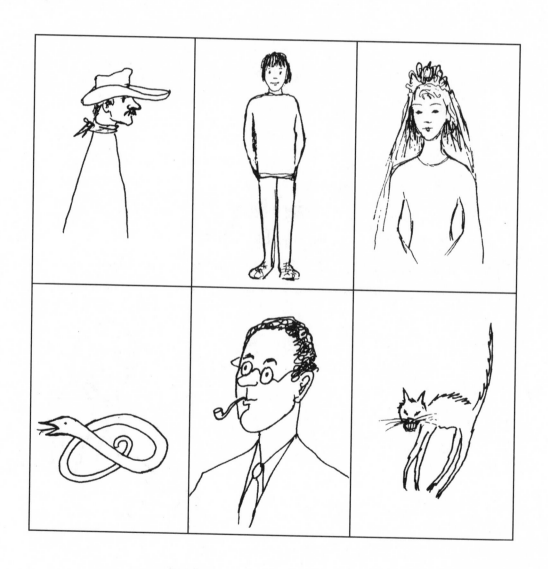

© 1983–2007 by Rawley Silver. Reprinted with permission for personal use only.

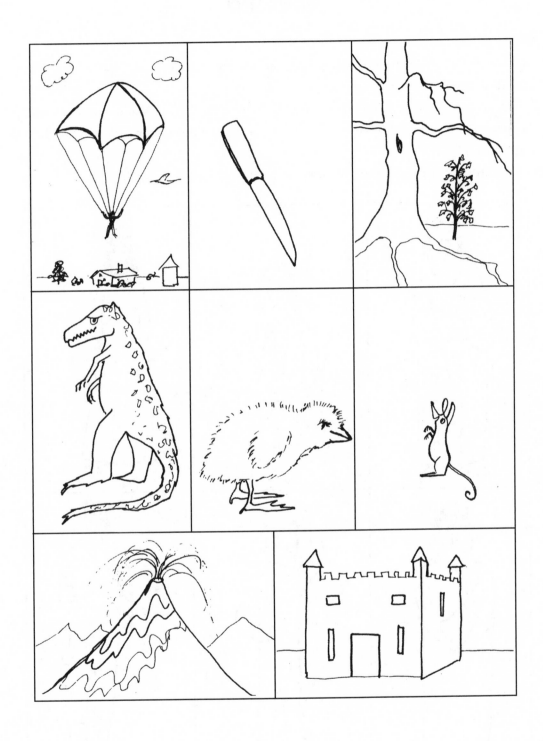

© 1983–2007 by Rawley Silver. Reprinted with permission for personal use only.

# Draw a Story

## Form B

Choose two of these drawings and imagine a story—something happening between the subjects you choose.

When you are ready, draw a picture of what you imagine. Make your drawing tell the story. Show what is happening. Feel free to change these drawings and to add your own ideas.

When you finish drawing, write the story in the place provided.

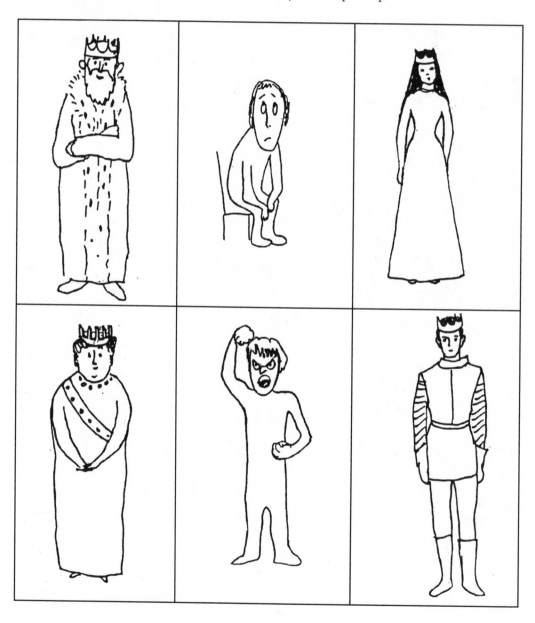

© 1983–2007 by Rawley Silver. Reprinted with permission for personal use only.

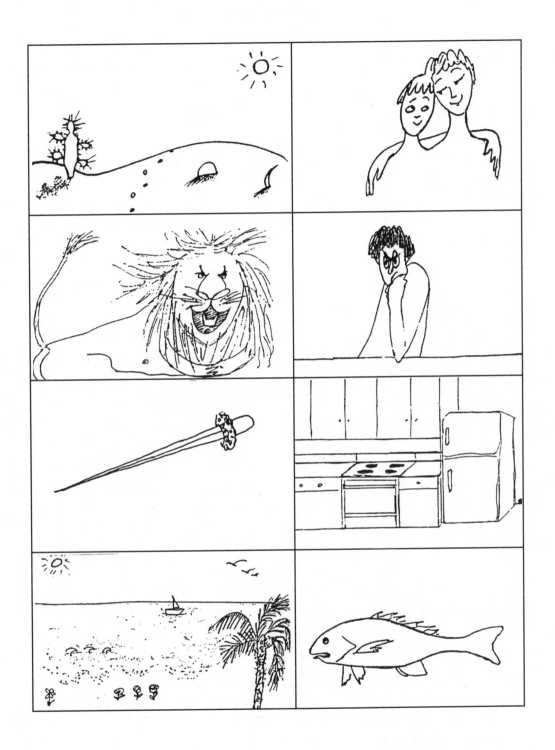

© 1983–2007 by Rawley Silver. Reprinted with permission for personal use only.

# Draw a Story

Drawing

Story:_____
_____
_____
_____
_____

Please fill in the blanks below:
First name ____ Sex____ Age ____ Location (state): _____ Date:_____
Just now I'm feeling ____very happy ____O.K. ____angry ____frightened ____sad

© 1983–2007 by Rawley Silver. Reprinted with permission for personal use only.

# Guidelines for Scoring Responses to the Draw a Story Assessment

## Scale for Assessing Emotional Content (Revised)

___1 point: strongly negative emotional content; for example:

    Solitary subjects who appear sad, helpless, isolated, suicidal, dead, or in mortal danger

    Relationships that appear life threatening or lethal

___2 points: moderately negative emotional content; for example:

    Solitary subjects that appear frightened, angry, frustrated, dissatisfied, worried, destructive, or unfortunate

    Relationships that appear stressful, hostile, destructive, or unpleasant

___2.5 points: ambiguous or ambivalent emotional content suggesting unpleasant or unfortunate outcomes

___3 points: ambiguous or ambivalent emotional content; for example, both negative and positive, neither negative nor positive, unemotional, or unclear

___3.5 points: ambiguous or ambivalent emotional content suggesting hopeful, pleasant, or fortunate outcomes

___4 points: moderately positive emotional content; for example:

    Solitary subjects who appear fortunate but passive

    Relationships that appear friendly or positive

___5 points: strongly positive emotional content; for example:

    Solitary subjects who appear happy, effective, or to be achieving goals

    Relationships that are caring or loving

© 2007 Rawley Silver.

## Scale for Assessing Self-Image (Revised)

___1 point: morbid self-image; respondent seems to identify with a subject who appears very sad, hopeless, helpless, isolated, suicidal, dead, or in mortal danger

___2 points: moderately negative self-image; respondent seems to identify with a subject who appears frightened, angry frustrated, dissatisfied, worried, or unfortunate

___2.5 points: unclear or ambivalent self-image with negative outcome; respondent seems to identify with a subject who appears unfortunate or likely to fail

___3 points: self-image is unclear, ambiguous, ambivalent, invisible, or absent

___3.5 points: unclear, ambivalent, or negative self-image, but outcome seems positive; respondent seems to identify with a subject who appears likely to achieve goal

___4 points: moderately positive self-image; respondent seems to identify with a subject who appears fortunate but passive, such as one who is watching television

___5 points: strongly positive self-image; respondent seems to identify with a subject who appears powerful, assaultive, intimidating, admirable, loved, or is achieving goals

© 2007 Rawley Silver.

## Scale for Assessing the Use of Humor

___1 point: lethal and morbid humor; for example:

    Amused by subject(s) dying painfully or in mortal danger and overtly expressing pain and/or fear, either through words or images

# Appendix B: Draw a Story

____1.5 points: lethal, but not morbid, humor; for example:

Amused by subject(s) disappearing, dead, or in mortal danger but not expressing pain and/or fear, either through words or images

____2 points: disparaging humor; for example:

Amused by a principal subject who is unlike the respondent (such as of the opposite gender) and unattractive, frustrated, foolish, or unfortunate, but not in mortal danger

____2.5 points: self-disparaging humor; for example:

Uses personal pronoun and/or is amused by a principal subject who is like the respondent as well as unattractive, frustrated, foolish, or unfortunate, but not in mortal danger

____3 points: ambiguous or ambivalent humor (neutral); for example:

Meaning or outcome is both negative and positive, neither negative nor positive, or unclear

____4 points: resilient humor (more positive than negative); for example:

Principal subject(s) overcome(s) adversity, or outcome is hopeful or favorable

____5 points: playful humor (entirely positive); for example:

Kindly, absurd, or playing on words, such as a rhyme or pun

## *Scales for Assessing Cognitive Skills*

### Ability to Select (Content or Meaning of the Response)

| | |
|---|---|
| 0 points | No evidence of selecting |
| 1 point | Perceptual level: single subject, or subjects unrelated in size or placement |
| 2 points | Subjects may be related in size or placement but there is no interaction |
| 3 points | Functional level: concrete, shows what subjects do, or what is done to them |
| 4 points | Descriptive rather than abstract or imaginative |
| 5 points | Conceptual level: imaginative, well-organized idea; implies more than is visible, or shows other ability to deal with abstract ideas |

### Ability to Combine (The Form of the Drawing)

| | |
|---|---|
| 0 points | Single subject, no spatial relationships |
| 1 point | Proximity: subjects float in space, related only by proximity |
| 2 points | Arrows, dotted lines, or other attempts to show relationships |
| 3 points | Baseline: subjects are related to one another along a baseline (real or implied) |
| 4 points | Beyond the baseline level, but much of the drawing area is blank |
| 5 points | Overall coordination; shows depth or takes into account the entire drawing area, or else includes a series of two or more drawings |

### Ability to Represent (Concepts and Creativity in the Form, Content, Title, or Story)

| | |
|---|---|
| 0 points | No evidence of representation |
| 1 point | Imitative: copies stimulus drawings or uses stick figures or stereotypes |
| 2 points | Beyond imitation, but drawing or ideas are commonplace |
| 3 points | Restructured: changes or elaborates on stimulus drawings or stereotypes |
| 4 points | Beyond restructuring: moderately original or expressive |
| 5 points | Transformational: highly original, expressive, playful, suggestive, or uses metaphors, puns, jokes, satire, or double meanings |

© 1995–2007 Rawley Silver.

# Record Sheet for Responses to the Draw a Story Assessment

Date _____
Administered by _____
Scored by _____
Institution _____

| ID or Name | Age | EC | S-I | Humor | Title | Notes |
|---|---|---|---|---|---|---|
| First Name | | | | | | |
| 1. | | | | | | |
| 2. | | | | | | |
| 3. | | | | | | |
| 4. | | | | | | |
| 5. | | | | | | |
| 6. | | | | | | |
| 7. | | | | | | |
| 8. | | | | | | |
| 9. | | | | | | |
| 10. | | | | | | |
| 11. | | | | | | |
| 12. | | | | | | |
| 13. | | | | | | |
| 14. | | | | | | |
| 15. | | | | | | |
| 16. | | | | | | |
| 17. | | | | | | |
| 18. | | | | | | |
| 19. | | | | | | |
| 20. | | | | | | |
| 21. | | | | | | |
| 22. | | | | | | |
| 23. | | | | | | |
| 24. | | | | | | |
| 25. | | | | | | |
| 26. | | | | | | |
| 27. | | | | | | |
| 28. | | | | | | |
| 29. | | | | | | |
| 30. | | | | | | |

Copyright 1987 Rawley Silver

## Appendix B: Draw a Story

# Results of the Draw a Story Assessment

Name: _____ Age: Sex: Date: _

School: _____ Administered by: _____

Subtest_____Pretest Norm _____

Score _____ Description  Score _____

Emotional Content

Self-Image

Use of Humor

Ability to Select

Ability to Combine

Creativity (Ability to Represent)

Subtest_____ Posttest Norm _____

Score _____Description __ Score ___

Emotional Content

Self-Image

Use of Humor

Ability to Select

Ability to Combine

Creativity (Ability to Represent)

Behaviors, Relationships, and/or Recommendations

_____

_____

_____

(use back of page for additional observations)

© 1983–2007 by Rawley Silver. Reprinted with permission for personal use only.

# Appendix C

# Stimulus Drawing Cards

◇    ◇    ◇

# Appendix C: Stimulus Drawing Cards

To remove cards, cut along solid outside lines, then cut cards apart.

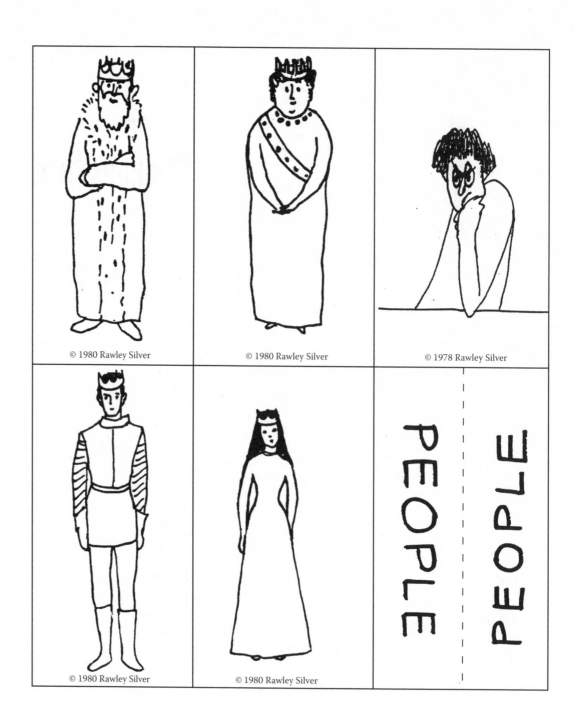

© 1980 Rawley Silver   © 1980 Rawley Silver   © 1978 Rawley Silver

© 1980 Rawley Silver   © 1980 Rawley Silver

## 1. Group A (People)

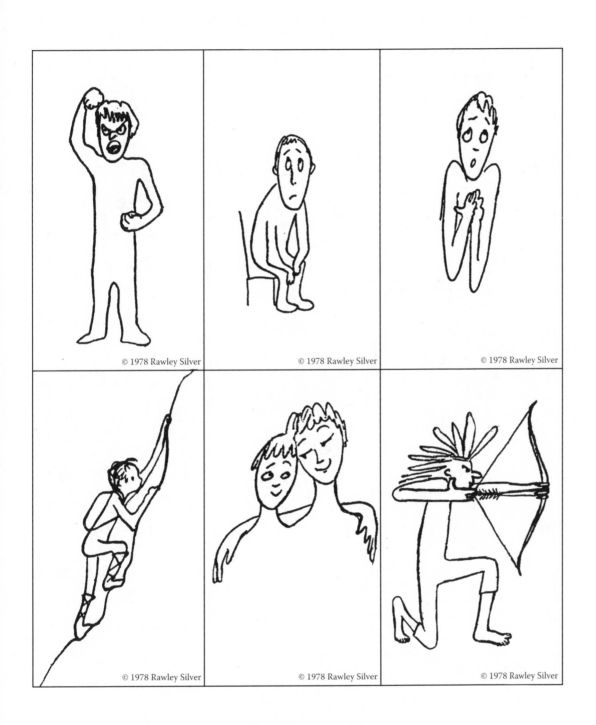

© 1978 Rawley Silver

© 1978 Rawley Silver

© 1978 Rawley Silver

© 1978 Rawley Silver

© 1978 Rawley Silver

© 1978 Rawley Silver

## 2. Group A (People)

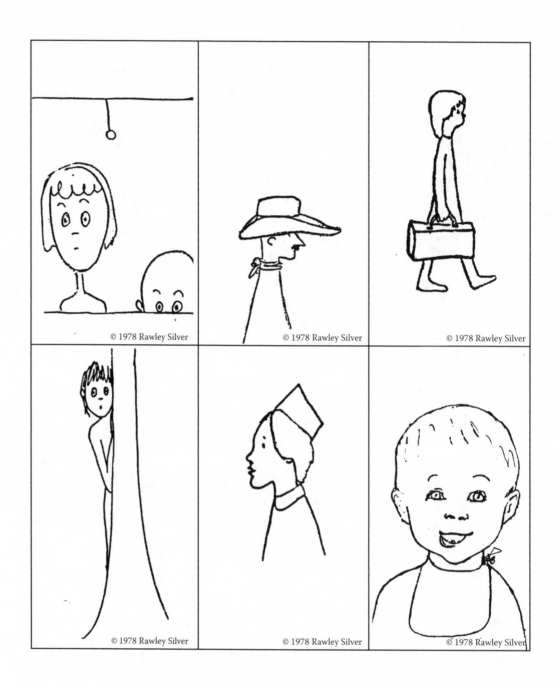

© 1978 Rawley Silver

© 1978 Rawley Silver

© 1978 Rawley Silver

© 1978 Rawley Silver

© 1978 Rawley Silver

© 1978 Rawley Silver

## 3. Group A (People)

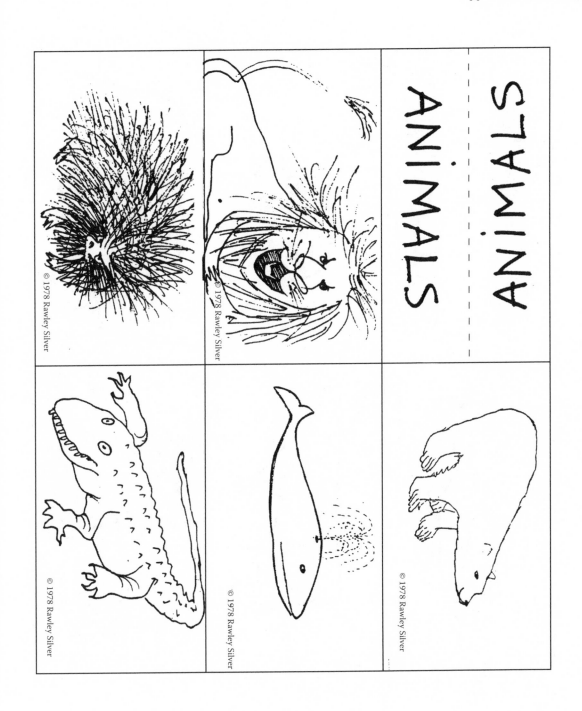

© 1978 Rawley Silver

## 4. Group B (Animals)

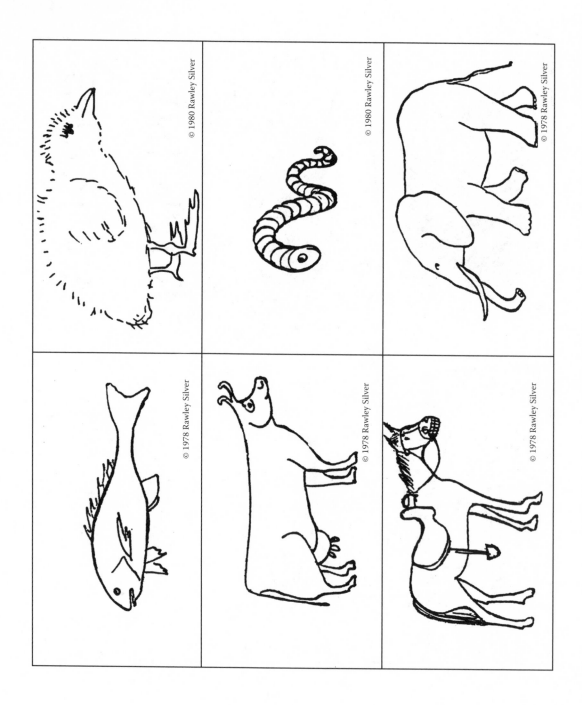

© 1980 Rawley Silver

© 1980 Rawley Silver

© 1978 Rawley Silver

© 1978 Rawley Silver

© 1978 Rawley Silver

© 1978 Rawley Silver

**5. Group B (Animals)**

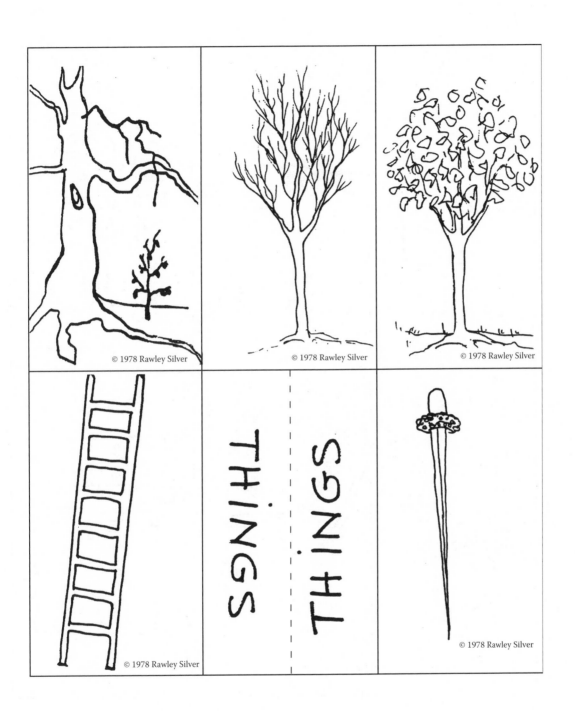

© 1978 Rawley Silver

© 1978 Rawley Silver

© 1978 Rawley Silver

© 1978 Rawley Silver

© 1978 Rawley Silver

## 6. Group C (Things)

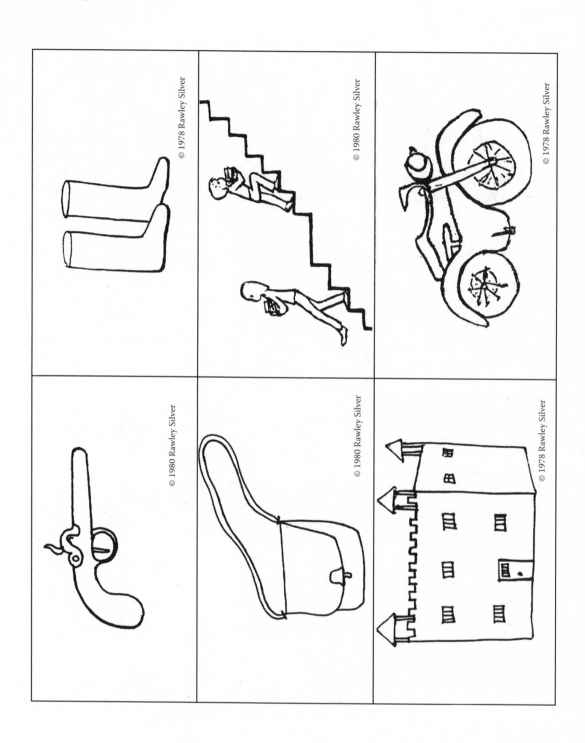

© 1978 Rawley Silver

© 1980 Rawley Silver

© 1978 Rawley Silver

© 1980 Rawley Silver

© 1980 Rawley Silver

© 1978 Rawley Silver

## 7. Group C (Things)

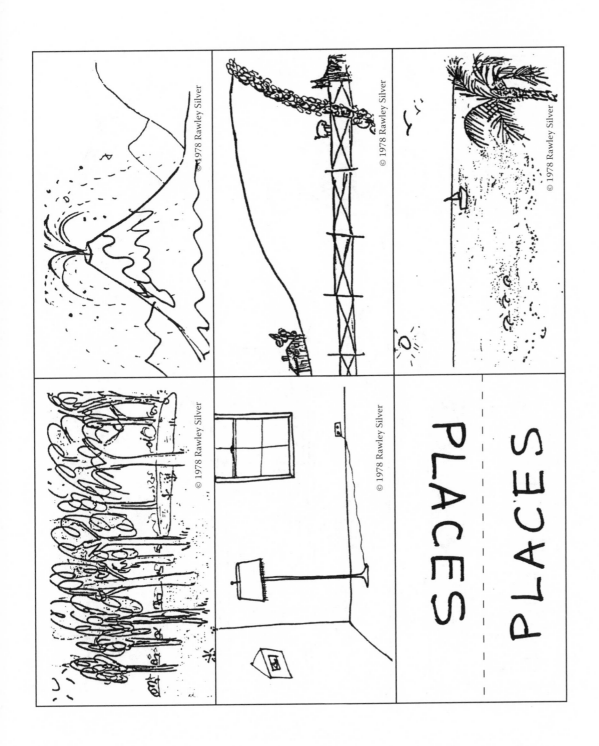

## 8. Group D (Places)

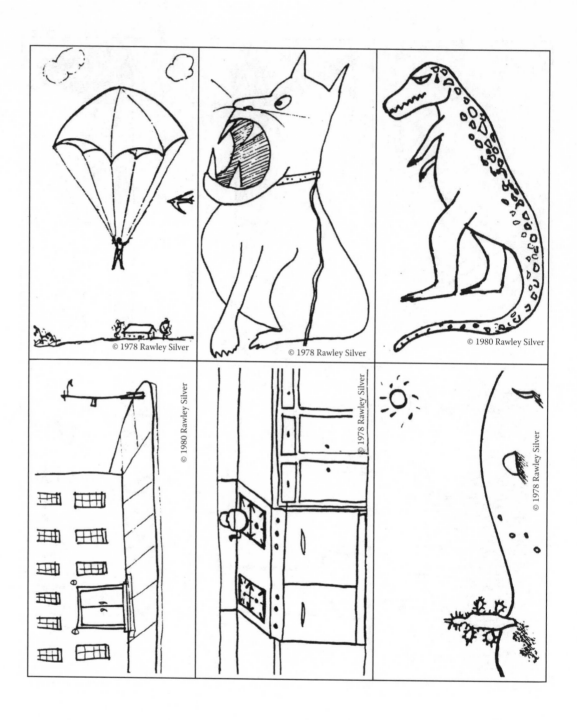

© 1978 Rawley Silver

© 1978 Rawley Silver

© 1980 Rawley Silver

© 1980 Rawley Silver

© 1978 Rawley Silver

© 1978 Rawley Silver

## 9. Group D (Places)

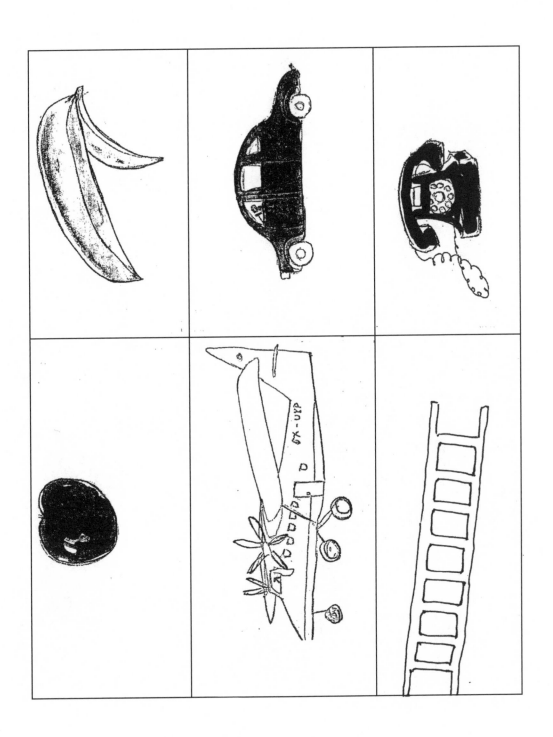

## 10. Group X (Food or Things)

# References

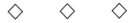

Allen, G. W. (1967). *William James*. New York: Viking.

Allessandrini, C. D., Duarte, J. L., Dupas, M. A., & Bianco, M. F. (1998). SDT: The Brazilian standardization of the Silver Drawing Test of Cognition and Emotion. *ARTherapy: Journal of the American Art Therapy Association, 15*(2), 107–115.

American Psychiatric Association (1994). *Diagnostic criteria from DSM-IV.* Washington, DC: Author.

Anderson, V. (2001). *A study of the correlations between the SDT Drawing from Imagination Subtest and the Gates-MacGinitie Reading Comprehension Test with middle school students.* Unpublished master's thesis, MCP Hahnemann University, Philadelphia.

Arnheim, R. (1969). *Visual thinking.* Berkeley and Los Angeles: University of California Press.

Bannatyne, A. (1971). *Language, reading, and learning disabilities.* Springfield, IL: Charles C Thomas.

Beck, A. T. (1978). *Depression inventory.* Philadelphia: Center for Cognitive Therapy.

Beck, A. T., Rush, J., Shaw, B. F., & Emory, G. (1979). *Cognitive theory of depression.* New York: Guilford Press.

Bjorkqvist, K., Osterman, K., & Kaukianen, A. (1992). The development of direct and indirect aggressive strategies in males and females. In K. Bjorkqvist & P. Niemela (Eds.). *Of mice and women: Aspects of female aggression.* San Diego, CA: Academic Press, cited in Connor, 2002.

# References

Blakeslee, S. (2006, January 10). Cells that read minds: A new look at mirror neurons. *New York Times*, p. D1.

Blasdel, L. (1997). *Critical thinking skills developed through visual art experiences.* Unpublished master's thesis, Emporia State University, Emporia, Kansas.

Bok, S. (1998). *Mayhem: Violence as public entertainment.* Brattleboro, VT: Perseus Books.

Bok, S. (2003). Study of happiness. *Newsday*, reprinted 11/23/03, *Sarasota Herald Tribune*.

Brandt, M. (1995). *Visual stories: A comparison study utilizing the Silver art therapy assessment with adolescent sex offenders.* Unpublished master's thesis, Ursuline College, Pepper Pike, Ohio.

Brenner, C. A. (1974). *Elementary textbook of psychoanalysis.* New York: Anchor.

Bronowski, J. (1973). *The ascent of man.* Boston: Little, Brown.

Bruner, J. S., Oliver, R. R., Greenfield, P. M., Hornsby, J. R., Kenny, H. J., Maccoby, M., et al. (Eds.). (1966). *Studies in cognitive growth.* New York: Wiley.

Buber, M. (1961). *Between man and man.* Boston: Beacon Press.

Buck, J. N. (1948). The H.T.P. technique: A qualitative and quantitative scoring method. *Journal of Clinical Psychology*, monograph no. 5.

Burns, R., & Kaufman, S. H. (1972). *Actions, styles, and symbols in kinetic family drawings.* New York: Brunner/Mazel.

California Achievement Tests (1957). Monterey, CA: CTB/McGraw-Hill.

Canadian Cognitive Abilities Test (1990). Scarboro, Ontario, Canada: Nelson.

Carrion, F., & Silver, R. (1991). Using the Silver Drawing Test in school and hospital. *American Journal of Art Therapy, 30*(2), 36–43.

Ching Hao. (1948). *The spirit of the brush* (S. Sakanishi, Trans.). London: John Murray.

Coffey, C. M. (1995). *Women, major depression, and imagery.* Unpublished master's thesis, Southern Illinois University, Edwardsville, Illinois.

Cohen, B. M. (1986). *The diagnostic drawing series.* Alexandria, VA: Author.

Connor, D. F. (2002). *Aggression and antisocial behavior in children and adolescents.* New York: Guilford Press.

Craig, H., & Gordon, H. (1989). Specialized cognitive function among deaf individuals; implications for instruction. In D. S. Martin (Ed.), *Cognition, education, and deafness.* Washington, DC: Gallaudet University Press.

Dalai Lama. (2005). *The universe in a single atom.* New York: Random House.

Damasio, A. R. (1994). *Descartes' error.* New York: Putnam.

Dhanachitsiriphong, P. (1999). *The effects of art therapy and rational emotive therapy on cognition and emotional development of male adolescents in Barn Karuna Training School of the Central Observation and Protection Center.* Unpublished master's thesis, Burapha University, Chonburi, Thailand.

Dunn-Snow, P. (1994). Adapting the Silver Draw a Story assessment: Art therapy techniques with children and adolescents. *American Journal of Art Therapy, 33* (November), 35–36.

Earwood, C., Fedorko, M., Holzman, E., Montanari, L., & Silver, R. (2004). Screening for aggression using the Draw a Story assessment. *ARTherapy: Journal of the American Art Therapy Association, 21*(3), 115–161.

Escobar, J. I. (1998). Why are immigrants better off? *Archives of General Psychiatry, 55*(9), 781–782.

Finney, P. (1994). A review of two art assessment tasks in an adult day treatment center. *ARTherapy: Journal of the American Art Therapy Association, 11*(2), 154–156.

Fischer, K., & Watson, M. (2002). Inhibited killers, *Harvard Magazine 104*(7) 12–13.

Fiske, E. B. (1999). *Champions of change. The impact of the arts on learning.* Washington, DC: The Arts Education Partnership; the President's Committee on Arts and the Humanities.

Fluornoy, E. (1995). In G. W. Allen, *William James.* New York: Viking.

Gallese, V., & Goldman, A. (1998). Mirror neurons and the simulation theory of mindreading. *Trends in Cognitive Sciences, 2*(12), 493–495.

Gallese, V., Keysers, C., & Rizzolatti, G. (2004). A unifying view of the basis of social cognition. *Trends in Cognitive Sciences, 8*(9), 396–403.

Gantt, L., & Tabone, C. (1998). *The formal elements art therapy scale: The rating manual.* Morgantown, WV: Gargoyle Press.

Gardner, H. (1993). *Multiple intelligences.* New York: Basic Books.

Gates-MacGinitie Reading Comprehension Test (1989). *Gates-MacGinitie Reading Comprehension Test, Evaluation 5–6, Form K., 7–9.* Itasca, IL: Riverside Press.

Gawanda, A. (2002). The learning curve. In O. Sacks (Ed.), *The best science writing, 2003* (pp. 49–67). New York: HarperCollins.

Gilligan, C., Ward, D., Taylor, J. M., & Bardige, B. (1988). *Mapping the moral domain.* Cambridge, MA: Harvard University Press.

Goodenough, F., & Harris, D. B. (1963). *Children's drawings as measures of mental maturity.* New York: Harcourt, Brace, and World.

Gur, C. (2006). *The effect of art education programs on drawing skills of six year old gifted children from high socio-economic status.* Unpublished doctoral dissertation, Gazi University, Ankara, Turkey.

Hayes, K. (1978). *The relationship between drawing ability and reading scores.* Unpublished master's thesis, College of New Rochelle, New Rochelle, New York.

Heath, W. (2000). Cancer comics: The humor of the tumor. *ArtTherapy: Journal of the American Art Therapy Association, 17*(1), 479.

Henn, K. (1990). *The effects of an integrated arts curriculum on the representation of spatial relationships.* Unpublished master's thesis, Buffalo State College, Buffalo, New York.

Hiscox, A. R. (1990). *An alternative to language-oriented IQ tests for learning-disabled children.* Unpublished master's thesis, College of Notre Dame, Belmont, California.

Hoffman, D. D. (1998). *Visual intelligence: How we create what we see.* New York: Norton.

Hornsby, J. J. (1966). On equivalence. In Bruner, Oliver, Greenfield, Hornsby, Kenny, Maccoby, et al. (Eds.), *Studies in cognitive growth* (pp. 79–85). New York: Wiley.

# References

Horovitz-Darby, E. (1991). Family art therapy within a deaf system. *Arts in Psychotherapy, 18*(3), 254–261.

Horovitz-Darby, E. (1996, November). Preconference presentation, Annual Conference of the American Art Therapy Association, Philadelphia.

Hunter, G. (1992). *An examination of some individual differences in information processing, personality, and motivation with respect to some dimensions of spatial thinking or problem solving in TAFE students.* Unpublished master's thesis, University of New England, Armidale, New South Wales, Australia.

Ione, A. (2000). Connecting the cerebral cortex with the artist's eyes, mind, and culture. *Journal of Consciousness Studies, 7*(8–9), 21–27.

Iowa Test of Basic Skills (2001). *Iowa Test of Basic Skills, form A.* Itasca, IL: Riverside.

Iowa Test of Basic Skills (2003). *Iowa Test of Basic Skills, form B.* Itasca, IL: Riverside.

Jakobson, R. (1964). Linguistic typology of aphasic impairment. In A. DeReuck & M. O'Conner (Eds.), *Disorder of language.* Boston: Little, Brown.

Jung, C. G. (1974). *Man and his symbols.* New York: Dell.

Kaplan, F. F. (2000). *Art, science, and art therapy.* London: Jessica Kingsley.

Koppitz, E. M. (1968). *Psychological evaluation of children's human figure drawings.* New York: Grune and Stratton.

Kopytin, A. (2002). The Silver Drawing Test of Cognition and Emotion: Standardization in Russia. *American Journal of Art Therapy, 40*(May), 223–237.

Kopytin, A., Svistovskaya, H., & Sventskaya, V. (2005). Cultural differences and similarities. In R. Silver (Ed.), *Aggression and depression assessed through art* (141–158). New York: Brunner-Routledge.

Kramer, E. (1971). *Art as therapy with children.* New York: Schocken Books.

Lachman-Chapin, M. (1987). M. Kohut's theories on narcissism: Implications for art therapy. *American Journal of Art Therapy, 19,* 3–9.

Lambert, C. (1999, September–October). *Harvard Magazine,* 46–53.

Lampart, M. T. (1960). The art work of deaf children. *American Annals of the Deaf, 105,* 419–423.

Lane, R. D., & Nadel, L. (2000). *Cognitive neuroscience of emotion.* New York: Oxford University Press.

Langer, S. K. (1957). *Problems of art.* New York: Scribner.

Langer, S. K. (1958). *Philosophy in a new key.* New York: Mentor Books.

Langer, S. K. (1962). *Reflections on art.* Baltimore: John Hopkins University Press.

LeDoux, J. (1996). *The emotional brain.* New York: Touchstone Books.

Levick, M. F. (1989). *The Levick Emotional and Cognitive Art Therapy Assessment (LECATA).* Miami: Author.

Linebaugh, A. J. (1996). *What the school age child perceives in a hospital environment: The DAS instrument with physically ill children.* Unpublished master's thesis, Long Island University, Brookville, New York.

MacNiel, G. (2002) School bullying: An overview. In L. Rapp-Paglicci, A. Roberts, & J. Wodarski (Eds.), *Handbook of violence.* New York: Wiley.

Malchiodi, C. A. (1997). *Breaking the silence.* New York: Brunner/Mazel.

Malchiodi, C. A. (1998). *Understanding children's drawings.* New York: Guilford Press.

Mango, C., & Richman, J. (1990). Humor and art therapy. *American Journal of Art Therapy 28*(May), 111–114.

Marshall, S. B. (1988). *The use of art therapy to foster cognitve skills with learning disabled children.* Unpublished master's thesis, Pratt Institute, Brooklyn, New York.

McGee, M. (1979). Human spatial abilities: Psychometric studies and environmental influences. *Psychological Bulletin, 86*(5), 889–918.

McKnew, H., Cytryn, L., & Yahries, H. (1983). *Why isn't Johnny crying?* New York: Norton.

Metropolitan Achievement Test (1993). San Antonio, TX: Harcourt Educational Measurement.

Metropolitan Reading Instructional Tests (1960). San Diego, CA: Psychological Corporation.

Miller, W. I. (1997). *The anatomy of disgust.* Cambridge, MA: Harvard University Press.

Moir, A., & Jessel, D. (1992). *Brain sex.* New York: Dell.

Moser, J. (1980). *Drawing and painting and learning disabilities.* Unpublished doctoral dissertation, New York University, New York.

Oliver, R. R., & Hornsby, J. R. (1966). On equivalence. In Bruner, J. S., Oliver, R. R., Greenfield, P. M., Hornsby, J. R., Kenny, H. J., Maccoby, M., et al. (Eds.), *Studies in cognitive growth* (pp. 79–85). New York: Wiley.

Otis-Lennon School Ability Test (2005). *Otis-Lennon School Ability Test* (8th ed.). San Antonio, TX: Harcourt Assessment.

Pannunzio, D. M. (1991). *Short-term adjunctive art therapy as a treatment intervention for depressed hospitalized youth.* Unpublished master's thesis, Ursuline College, Pepper Pike, Ohio.

Pfeffer, C. R. (1986). *The suicidal child.* New York: Guilford Press.

Pfeiffer, L. J. (2005). Foreword. In R. Silver (Ed.), *Aggression and depression assessed through art.* New York: Brunner-Routledge.

Piaget, J. (1970). *Genetic epistemology.* New York: Columbia University Press.

Piaget, J., & Inhelder, B. (1967). *The child's conception of space.* New York: Norton.

Polio, H. R. & Polio, M. R. (1992). Current research in cognition, education, and deafness: Some observations from a different point of view. In D. S. Martin (Ed.), *Cognition, education, and deafness.* Washington, DC: Gallaudet University Press.

Ramachandran, V. S., & Hirstein, W. (1999). The science of art: A neurological theory of aesthetic experience. *Journal of Consciousness Studies, 6*(6–7), 15–51.

Restak, R. M. (1994). *The modular brain.* New York: Scribner.

Rubin, J. A. (1987). *Approaches to art therapy.* New York: Brunner/Mazel.

Rubin, J. A. (1999). *Art therapy: An introduction.* New York: Brunner/Mazel.

Rugel, R. P. (1974). WISC subtest scores of disabled readers: A review. *Journal of Learning Disabilities, 7,* 57–64.

# References

Sandburg, L., Silver, R., & Vilstrup, K. (1984). The stimulus drawing technique with adult psychiatric patients, stroke patients, and adolescents in art therapy. *ARTherapy: Journal of the American Art Therapy Association, 1*(3), 132–140.

Schaffer, D., & Fisher, P. (1981). The epidemiology of suicide in children and young adolescents. *Journal of the American Academy of Child Psychiatry, 21*, 545–565.

Schlain, L. (1998). *The alphabet versus the goddess.* New York: Penguin.

Shoemaker, R. (1977). The significance of the first picture in art therapy. In *The Dynamics of Creativity. Proceedings of the 8th annual conference of the American Art Therapy Association.* Baltimore, MD: AATA Publications Committee.

Silver, R. (1962). Potentialities in art education for the deaf. *Eastern Arts Quarterly, 1*(2), 30–38.

Silver, R. (1963). Art for the deaf child: Its potentialities. *Volta Review, 65*(8), 408–413.

Silver, R. (1966). The role of art in the conceptual thinking, adjustment, and aptitudes of deaf and aphasic children (Doctoral dissertation, Columbia University, 1966). *Dissertation Abstracts International,* no. 66-8230.

Silver, R. (1967). *A demonstration project in art education for deaf and hard of hearing children and adults.* U.S. Office of Education, Bureau of Research Project #6-8598. (ERIC Document Reproduction Service No. ED013009)

Silver, R. (1971). The role of art in the cognition, adjustment, transfer, and aptitudes of deaf children. In C. Deussen (Ed.), *Proceedings of the Conference on Art for the Deaf* (pp. 15–26). Los Angeles: Junior Art Center.

Silver, R. (1972). *The transfer of cognition and attitudes of deaf and aphasic children through art.* Springfield: State of Illinois, Office of the Superintendent of Public Instruction.

Silver, R. (1973). *A study of cognitive skills development through art experiences.* New York City Board of Education, New York State Urban Education Project No. 147-232-101. (ERIC Document Reproduction Service No. ED084745, EC060575)

Silver, R. (1975a). Children with communication disorders: Cognitive and artistic development. *American Journal of Art Therapy, 14*(2), 39–47.

Silver, R. (1975b). Clues to cognitive functioning in the drawings of stroke patients. *American Journal of Art Therapy, 15*(10), 3–8.

Silver, R. (1975c). Using art to evaluate and develop cognitive skills. Paper presented at the Annual Conference of the American Art Therapy Association. (ERIC Document Reproduction Service No. ED116401, EC080793)

Silver, R. (1976a). *Shout in silence: Visual arts and the deaf.* Exhibition catalog. New York: Metropolitan Museum of Art.

Silver, R. (1976b). Using art to evaluate and develop cognitive skills: Children with communication disorders and children with learning disabilities. *American Journal of Art Therapy, 16*(1), 11–19.

Silver, R. (1977). The question of imagination, originality, and abstract thinking by deaf children. *American Annals of the Deaf, 122*(3), 349–354. (ERIC Document Reproduction Service No. ED166043, EC093422)

Silver, R. (1978). *Developing cognitive and creative skills through art.* Baltimore: University Park Press.

Silver, R. (1979). *Art as language for the handicapped.* Exhibition catalog. Washington, DC: Smithsonian Institution. (ERIC Document Reproduction Service No. ED185774)

Silver, R. (1982a). *Stimulus drawings and techniques in therapy, development, and assessment.* New York: Trillium Books.

Silver, R. (1982b). Developing cognitive skills through art. In L. G. Katz (Ed.), *Current topcs in early childhood education* (Vol. 4, pp. 143–171). Norwood, NJ: Ablex. (ERIC Document Reproduction Service No. ED207674)

Silver, R. A. (1983a). Identifying gifted handicapped children through their drawings. *ARTherapy: Journal of the American Art Therapy Association, 1*(10), 40–46. (ERIC Document Reproduction Service No. EJ295217)

Silver, R. (1983b). *Silver Drawing Test of Cognition and Emotion.* Seattle, WA: Special Child Publications.

Silver, R. (1986). *Stimulus drawings and techniques in therapy, development, and assessment.* New York: Trillium Books.

Silver, R. (1987a). A cognitive approach to art therapy. In J. Rubin (Ed.), *Approaches to art therapy* (pp. 233–250). New York: Brunner/Mazel.

Silver, R. (1987b). Sex differences in the emotional content of drawings. *ARTherapy: Journal of the American Art Therapy Association, 4*(2), 67–77.

Silver, R. (1988a). Screening children and adolescents for depression through Draw a Story. *American Journal of Art Therapy, 26*(4) 119–124.

Silver, R. (1988b). Draw a Story: Screening for depression. Mamaroneck, NY: Ablin Press.

Silver, R. (1989a). *Developing cognitive and creative skills through Art.* Mamaroneck, New York: Ablin Press. (ERIC Document Reproduction Service No. 410 479)

Silver, R. (1989b). *Stimulus drawings and techniques in therapy, development, and assessment.* New York: Trillium Books.

Silver, R. (1990). *The Silver Drawing Test of Cognition and Emotion* (2nd ed.). Sarasota, FL: Ablin Press.

Silver, R. (1991). *Stimulus drawings and techniques in therapy, development, and assessment* (3rd ed.). Sarasota, FL: Ablin Press.

Silver, R. (1992). Gender differences in drawings: A study of self-images, autonomous subjects, and relationships. *ARTherapy: Journal of the American Art Therapy Association, 9*(2), 85–92.

Silver, R. (1993a). Age and gender differences expressed through drawings: A study of attitudes toward self and others. *ARTherapy: Journal of the American Art Therapy Association, 10*(3), 159–168.

Silver, R. (1993b). Assessing the emotional content of drawings by older adults. *American Journal of Art Therapy, 32*, 46–52.

# References

Silver, R. (1993c). *Draw a Story: Screening for depression and age or gender differences.* New York: Trillium Press.

Silver, R. (1996a). Gender differences and similarities in the spatial abilities of adolescents. *ARTherapy: Journal of the American Art Therapy Association, 13*(2), 118–120. (ERIC Document Reproduction Service No. EJ530390)

Silver, R. (1996b). Sex differences in the solitary and assaultive fantasies of delinquent and non-delinquent adolescents. *Adolescence, 31*(123), 543–552.

Silver, R. (1996c). *The Silver Drawing Test of Cognition and Emotion* (3rd ed.). Sarasota, FL: Ablin Press.

Silver, R. (1997a). Sex and age differences in attitudes toward the opposite sex. *ARTherapy: Journal of the American Art Therapy Association, 14*(4), 268–272.

Silver, R. (1997b). *Stimulus drawings and techniques in therapy, development, and assessment* (5th ed.). Sarasota, FL: Ablin Press.

Silver, R. (1998a). Gender parity and disparity in spatial skills: Comparing horizontal, vertical, and other task performances. *ARTherapy: Journal of the American Art Therapy Association, 15*(1), 38–46.

Silver, R. (1998b). *Updating the Silver Drawing Test and Draw a Story manuals.* Sarasota, FL: Ablin Press.

Silver, R. (1999). Differences among aging and young adults in attitudes and cognition. *ARTherapy: Journal of the American Art Therapy Association, 16*(3), 133–139.

Silver, R. (2000a). *Developing cognitive and creative skills through art: Programs for children with communication disorders* (4th ed.). Lincoln, NE: iUniverse.

Silver, R. (2000b). *Draw a Story: Screening for depression and age or gender differences.* Sarasota, FL: Ablin Press.

Silver, R. (2000c). *Studies in art therapy (1962–2000).* Sarasota, FL: Ablin Press.

Silver, R. (2001). *Art as language: Access to emotions and cognitive skills.* New York: Brunner-Routledge.

Silver, R. (2002). *Three art assessments: The Silver Drawing Test of Cognition and Emotion, Draw a Story: Screening for Depression; and Stimulus Drawings and Techniques.* New York: Brunner-Routledge.

Silver, R. (2003). *Humorous responses to a drawing task, ranging from lethal to playful.* Washington, DC: U.S. Department of Education (ERIC Document Reproduction Service No. ED474679, CG032289)

Silver, R. (Ed.). (2005). *Aggression and depression assessed through art: Using Draw a Story to identify children and adolescents at risk.* New York: Brunner-Routledge.

Silver, R., Boeve, E., Hayes, K., Itzler, J., Lavin, C., O'Brien, J., et al. (1980). *Assessing and developing cognitive skills in handicapped children through art.* National Institution of Education Project No. G790081. College of New Rochelle, New Rochelle, New York. (ERIC Document Reproduction Service No. ED209878)

Silver, R., & Carrion, F. (1991). Using the *Silver Drawing Test* in school and hospital. *American Journal of Art Therapy, 30*(2), 36–43.

Silver, R., & Ellison, J. (1995). Identifying and assessing self-images in drawings by delinquent adolescents. *Arts in Psychotherapy, 22*(4), 339–352. (ERIC Document Reproduction Service No. EJ545763)

Silver, R., & Lavin, C. (1977). The role of art in developing and evaluating cognitive skills. *Journal of Learning Disabilities, 10*(7), 416–424. (ERIC Document Reproduction Service No. ED101654, EJ171839)

Sinclair-de-Zwart, H. (1969). Developmental psycholinguistics. In Elkin, D., & Flavel, J. H. (Eds.), *Studies in cognitive development.* London: Oxford University Press.

Sless, D. S. (1981). *Learning and visual communication.* New York: Wiley.

Smith, M. D., Coleman, J. J., Dokecki, P. R., & Davis, E. E. (1977). Intellectual characteristics of school labeled learning disabled children. *Exceptional Child, 4*(6), 352–357.

Sonstroem, A. M. (1996). On the conservation of solids. In Bruner, J. S., Oliver, R. R., Greenfield, P. H., Hornsby, J. R., Kenny, H. J., Maccoby, M., et al. (Eds.), *Studies in cognitive growth.* New York: Wiley.

SRA Reading Achievement Test and Survey of Basic Skills Ability (1978). McMillan-McGraw-Hill. Monterey, CA.

Stern, C. (1965). *The flight from woman.* New York: Noonday Press.

Sternberg, R. J. (1997). *Successful intelligence.* New York: Plume.

Tannen, D. (1990). *You just don't understand.* New York: Ballantine Books.

Tinen, L. (1990). Biological processes in nonverbal communication and their role in the making and interpretation of art. *American Journal of Art Therapy, 29*(8), 9–13.

Torrance, E. P. (1962). *Guiding creative talent.* Englewood Cliffs, NJ: Prentice Hall.

Torrance, E. P. (1980). Creative intelligence and an agenda for the 80s. *Art Education, 33*(7), 8–14.

Torrance, E. P. (1984). *The Torrance Test of Creative Thinking, Figural Form A.* Bensonville, IL: Scholastic Testing Service.

Turner, C. (1993). Draw a Story in the assessment of abuse. Preconference presentation, 1993 Annual Conference of the American Art Therapy Association, Atlanta.

Ulman, E. (1987). *Ulman Personality Assessment Procedure.* Montpelier, VT: American Journal of Art Therapy.

Vaillard, G. (2002) *Aging well.* Boston: Little, Brown, and Company.

Vega, W. A., Kolody, B., Aguilar-Gaxiola, S., Alderete, E., Catalano, R., & Caraveo-Anduaga, J. (1998). Lifetime prevalence of DSM-III-R psychiatric disorders among urban and rural Mexican Americans in California. *Archives of General Psychiatry, 55*(9), 771–780.

Wadeson, H. (1980). *Art psychotherapy.* New York: Wiley.

Wechsler, D. (1997). *Wechsler Adult Intelligence Scale* (3rd ed.). San Antonio, TX: PsychCorp.

Wechsler, D. (2003). *Wechsler Intelligence Scale for Children* (4th ed.). San Antonio, TX: PsychCorp.

# References

Whitehurst, G. (1984). Interrater agreement for journal manuscript reviews. *American Psychologist, 39,* 22–28.

White-Wolff, E. (1991). *Art and sand play in twins.* Unpublished master's thesis, Sonoma State University, Rohmert Park, California.

Williams, F. E. (1980). *Creativity Assessment Packet.* Buffalo, NY: DOK.

Wilson, M. F. (1990). *Art therapy as an adjunctive treatment modality with depressed hospitalized adolescents.* Unpublished master's thesis, Ursuline College, Pepper Pike, Ohio.

Wilson, M. F. (1993). Assessment of brain injury patients with the Draw a Story instrument. Preconference presentation, 1993 Annual Conference of the American Art Therapy Association, Atlanta.

Winder, B. W. (1962). *Statistical principles in experimental design.* New York: McGraw-Hill.

Witkin, H. A. (1962). *Psychological differentiation.* New York: John Wiley.

Zeki, S. (1999). *Inner vision: An exploration of art and the brain.* Oxford: Oxford University Press.

Zeki, S. (2001). Artistic creativity and the brain. *Science, 293*(July), 51.

Ziv, A. (1984). *Personality and sense of humor.* New York: Springer.

# Index

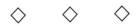

# Index

# Index

# Index